RESCUE 911

TALES FROM A FIRST RESPONDER

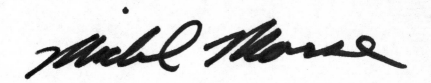

MICHAEL MORSE

Post Hill
PRESS

RESCUE 911

TALES FROM INCIDENT RESPONSE

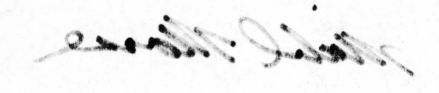

MICHAEL MORSE

Also by Michael Morse

Rescuing Providence
Rescue 1 Responding
City Life

A POST HILL PRESS BOOK
ISBN: 978-1-68261-286-6
ISBN (eBook): 978-1-68261-287-3

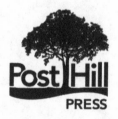

Post Hill Press
New York • Nashville
posthillpress.com

Published in the United States of America

To MSG Robert Morse,

43rd Military Police Brigade, US Army

ACKNOWLEDGMENTS

Thanks to Ben Pugh, Lauren Carter, Rebecca Violet, and Joe McCue at Uniform Stories, Greg Friese at EMS 1, Diane Rothschild at *Fire Engineering*, and Nancy Perry at *EMS World* for seeing the value in my work and publishing my stories. Thank you for sharing the message and promoting the good work that firefighters, paramedics, EMTs, and police officers do, day in and day out.

FOREWORD

Back in 2009, I discovered a blog called *Rescuing Providence*. The author, a lieutenant with the Providence, Rhode Island, Fire Department, had a gift for capturing the drudgery, drama, humor, and pathos of EMS, and I soon bought the book of the same name, a chronicle of one thirty-four-hour shift on Rescue 1 in Providence. I read it in one sitting, immediately realizing that, in comparison, I still had much growing to do as a writer and storyteller. Thus was my introduction to Michael Morse.

In the genre of EMS memoirs and fiction, there are two types of authors: paramedics who write about what they do, and writers who work on an ambulance as their full-time jobs. Discerning between the two is as easy as reading their work. Michael Morse is that second type. His prose is spare, often terse, but wonderfully descriptive. In a genre where most offerings are the EMS equivalent of a Faulkner novel, long and rambling but without the elegance of craft, Michael Morse is a Hemingway. He is able to wring more humanity out of a short, declarative sentence than most of us can in a paragraph, myself included. Michael Morse is simply a better storyteller than I.

Like *Rescuing Providence* before it, *Rescue 911: Tales from a First Responder* chronicles Morse's days at the Providence Fire Department in a series of short vignettes, each capturing something memorable about the encounter. He captures every element of a career spent as a caregiver: the fear, the drudgery, the system abuse, the boring routine, the triumph and the tragedy, the sublime and the silly. He offers a stark and unsparing glimpse into the life of an EMT, with none of the "Look at me, I'm a hero!" melodrama so common in EMS memoirs. Instead, Michael Morse pens a love song to our profession by simply showing you what EMS is, without glamor. He affords you a window into humanity, raw and real, and trusts the reader to make the judgment as to whether the profession, and those practicing it, acquits themselves with honor.

In the pages of this book, I think you'll see that they do.

Kelly Grayson,
Author of *En Route:*
A Paramedic's Stories of Life,
Death, and Everything In Between

INTRODUCTION

"Welcome to Providence," my training officer said to us, sixty-four trainees all about to begin a career in the fire service. Some of us had experience, some did not. We were told to forget everything we knew or thought we knew about the vocation we had chosen, because now we were going to learn things "the Providence way."

Most of us made it out of the academy, and many of those who did made it another twenty years and retired. Some were injured and had to leave before they were ready, some of us are still working twenty-five years later. New faces are introduced every few years, trainees become probies, probies become firefighters, firefighters become officers, and some of those become chiefs.

One thing remains certain: every person who raises their right hand and takes the oath of office is from that day forward until the day they die a firefighter. While never forgetting who we were before, we know that we will never be the same. It is an honor to belong in the fire service, not because of who we are as individuals, rather because of those who came before us, and wore the uniform well, worked, lived and sometimes died doing the job.

At the end of the day, when the smoke has cleared, and the fires are out, and we make it home, we can rest easy, knowing that others like us are on duty, keeping things safe. We know this because we live it, every second of every day, for life.

Magic

We're driving down Angel Street at three o'clock in the afternoon, perfect late summer day, nice iced coffee in the cup holder, pretty girls in summer dresses everywhere and no runs coming our way. We approach the Rhode Island School of Design just as a bus is leaving, full of kids going home from a weeklong summer program.

The bus is packed, and it slowly pulls away from the school ready to bring the kids back to wherever it is they came from. I hear shouting behind us, a happy sound, kids whooping it up. Dozens run past us, flanking the bus, jumping up and down, waving, smiling from ear to ear. The kids in the bus respond in kind, and it is sweet mayhem for a minute, then the bus moves down the hill, toward the city.

The spontaneous honor guard follows, escorting the bus, shouting, waving, keeping pace for a while before the machinery outpaces the humans and distance spreads. The guard keeps running. They catch the bus at the next light, more euphoria ensues, the joyous cacophony contagious as pedestrians and drivers, and tired EMTs, are caught up in the display of affection and sheer, unblemished happiness.

A few join in and honk their horns, or raise their hands in the air, or chirp their siren and the bus moves again, finally outdistancing the pack. The tired runners slow down, then stop, then turn around and head back up the hill and wait for their bus to take them back to wherever it is they come from, new friendships formed, and an experience that will last them a lifetime.

I'm stunned at the effect this little moment of magic has on me. The drowned two-year-old, the dead twenty-five-year-old, the beaten teen, the hopeless and lost all recede into the back of my mind and light shines through. It is a moment of grace delivered at just the right time and I never saw it coming, or knew how badly I needed it.

A call came in, we had to respond, and my voice sounded a little different when I answered the radio, and wiped my eyes, knowing that no matter what, things will be all right.

Numbers

Wind, gritty with sand lifted from the pavement, pecked at the skin on our faces, bitter, painful, and relentless.

"Come with me, it's freezing out here," I said to the woman. She stared into the wind, unblinking. Tears rolled down her face, she made no effort to wipe them away.

"Come on now, we can't leave you here," I said, taking hold of her coat. It was a nice one, hardly used.

"There's cats in the meadow," she said, and followed me.

"Are there, and what kind of cats might they be?"

She made eye contact then, and continued.

"The bisque is frozen, better get on with it then."

"You can't eat frozen bisque."

"The pencils need sharpening."

"I hate writing with dull pencils. Do you write often?"

"If the laundry is done in time, we'll go to the park."

"Is the park near your home?"

Nothing then, but at least we were inside the rescue, heading toward Rhode Island Hospital and safety. She had been wandering around downtown for hours, and nobody paid her any attention. The city is full of strange characters, she mixed in with the rest, and appeared to belong.

"Where do you live?"

Nothing.

"I bought a lottery ticket yesterday, 423-5342."

She looked up, and again made eye contact.

"476-2343."

She stayed interested.

"942-8725."

She continued staring, but spoke.

"2372983. 2372983. 2372983."

I wrote the number down. When we pulled into the rescue bay at the hospital. I used the truck phone and dialed the number. It hadn't rung once when a frantic voice picked up.

"Hello."

"This is Lieutenant Morse with the Providence Fire Department."

"Oh my God, is she okay?"

"I have a woman here, mid-sixties, nicely dressed and appears lost."

"Where are you?"

"Rhode Island Hospital."

"Where?"

"Rhode Island Hospital."

"Is her name Ruth?"

I looked at the woman, who was gone again.

"Ruth!"

She didn't budge, or respond.

"I don't know, she has no ID, but is wearing a black velvet coat with fur trim on the collar."

"That's her, thank you so much, we'll be there as soon as we can. It's an hour drive from Massachusetts."

"Massachusetts?"

"She likes buses."

An hour later Ruth was reunited with her daughter, son-in-law, five of six kids, and a few other people. She had been missing for sixteen hours. She had been diagnosed with Alzheimer's just this year. I have no idea what possessed me to start running off numbers. I guess I figured something in her mind might click.

I've done a lot of things over the last twenty years, but that call was one of the most gratifying moments of my career. The family treated me like a hero, and asked again and again how I got her to come up with the phone number. Truth is, I just got lucky.

A woman suffering from dementia was found dead in a ditch in Newport last week. She wandered off. Before she was found I heard a press release saying she liked to sit on public benches. I looked, but never saw her.

What's the Worst That Could Happen?

"I need a shower, think I have time?"

"What's the worst that could happen?" I answered.

Ed was working overtime and wanted a fresh start to the day. I was filling in for a rescue officer who was off on an injury. It was my first experience in charge of a fire department vehicle. Rescue 3 is quartered at the Branch Avenue Fire Station. It is a workhorse; five thousand runs annually the norm. All of Providence's advanced life support vehicles are workhorses, the call volume dramatically increasing as the years progress.

"Keep your radio on in case we get a call," I said as the door to the shower room closed.

This should have been my first day back on Engine 9 after a six-month detail to the rescue division. I enjoyed my time on Rescue 1, learned a lot and considered going back eventually, but I missed the camaraderie at the fire station and, of course, the firefighting. Providence rescues still respond to fires but for the most part stay outside and tend to the wounded.

I was looking forward to the old routine, the discussion around the coffee pot, the housework, polishing brass, checking the trucks, rechecking the trucks, making lunch and, with any luck, fighting a little of the red devil.

I didn't get a chance to walk in the door of the Brook Street Fire Station.

"Welcome back, Morse, you're going to Rescue 3, in charge," said Tim, my truck mate from Engine 9, from the second-floor kitchen window.

"See you tomorrow," he said, laughing, and shut the window so as not to let the cool air from the air conditioner out. I didn't take it personally; I knew Tim was looking forward to my return, we got along pretty well. I would just have to wait another day.

I knew there was a possibility of being sent back to the rescue but I didn't think it would happen so fast. The division is in desperate need of bodies. Not many firefighters are willing to be permanently assigned to the little white truck when the big red one is available. I put my gear back in the wagon and started toward the Branch Avenue fire barn and Rescue 3.

The shower water must not have had a chance to get hot when the bell tipped.

"Rescue 3 and Engine 2; respond to I-95 North for an accident involving a school bus."

Great.

"Rescue 3, responding."

I heard Engine 2 roar out of the station. Thirty seconds later, Ed appeared from the shower, soaking wet and getting dressed while walking toward the stairs.

"What's the worst that could happen?" he said, shaking his head.

"I should know better," I responded as the overhead door let the warm summer air into the bay. There are certain things that should never be uttered when on the clock. It's quiet. Things are so peaceful. What's the worst that could happen?

"Engine 2 to fire alarm, we have a school bus into a tractor trailer, heavy damage to the school bus. We'll keep you informed."

"Here we go," I said to Ed as we sped toward the incident.

"Engine 2 to fire alarm, advise rescue we have a pediatric trauma code, expedite."

The school bus driver drifted from her lane of travel at just the wrong time. A flatbed truck had stopped in the breakdown lane. The bus slammed into it, first smashing the windshield glass, then tearing into the passenger compartment, ripping the metal like a tin can. The baby didn't have a chance. She was in an infant seat at the door when the back of the flatbed crashed into the passenger compartment.

We approached from the south. The roof of the bus was torn off the body three quarters down the passenger side. I saw another Providence rescue just ahead of the bus. Brian took a bloody, still infant away from a woman who had stopped to help and started CPR.

The mind has a way of slowing things down during crisis. In what seemed slow motion, Ed pulled Rescue 3 past the wreckage while I assessed the situation from the officer's seat. I fully expected mangled bodies of school kids inside the bus. The bus appeared empty when I looked through the shattered windows. The truck stopped, I stepped out and approached the wreckage, not really prepared for what lay inside but forging ahead anyway. The driver of the bus sat slumped over the wheel, trapped. Another woman was trapped in the seat behind the driver. I forced myself to look down the narrow corridor for more victims. There were none. The bus had finished its morning route and was headed back to the garage.

Special Hazards arrived on scene and began extrication procedures. The state police blocked the highway while we worked. I watched the firefighters work like madmen during the extrication. I felt helpless standing on the highway, waiting. Fifteen minutes into the operation the infant's mother was freed from her temporary prison. We lifted her out, using the freshly opened roof of the bus as an extrication route. She was unconscious, in shock, and had deformities to her extremities. We got her into the rescue and rolled toward Rhode Island Hospital, the area's Level 1 Trauma Center, about ten minutes away. She lived. Her baby did not.

"What's the worst that could happen?"

Don't ask.

And so began the second part of my career in the fire service. I'm still a firefighter; once a person experiences that life it never leaves, it's in your blood. For now, I spend my time on the rescue, EMS a second calling. I got off to a rough start, and the road hasn't gotten much easier to travel, but for all the pain, lost sleep, and time away from my family, I can't imagine doing anything else.

Heartbeat

The kid was alive when Engine 3 arrived, but died within minutes.

"Engine 3 to fire alarm, eleven-year-old male, code 99."

"Rescue 1, received."

I put the mic down and put on the gloves. My new partner, Adam, picked up the pace, instinctively knowing this was the real thing. We arrived on scene thirty seconds later, entered the home, and saw CPR in progress.

"He was breathing when we got here, then he stopped and went pulseless."

We put him on a backboard, continued CPR, picked up our equipment and patient, and carried him out of his home, through a snow squall and into the rescue. His mother sat in the front, peering back as we worked. The monitor showed asystole, no shock advised. Joe worked like a madman trying to find a vein while Donna and Adam did CPR.

"What medical condition does he have," I asked his mother, trying to keep my voice steady.

"A neurological disorder that causes seizures. He was at the doctor's today for trouble breathing."

She sounded calm, I think she was in shock. Joe found a good vein and sank the IV.

"Go," I said to Ray, a new guy who was in the driver's seat. He sped toward Hasbro while we continued to work. One round of epi; pulseless. We tried an atropine; nothing. I attempted to tube him, the potholes made it difficult, I failed then picked up the phone.

"Rescue 1 to Hasbro, I've got an asystolic eleven-year-old male, CPR in progress, IV established, ETA two minutes."

The doctor on the other end of the phone asked a few questions. I gave the answers best I could, then hung up the phone. Another round of epi was ineffective. We brought him into the ER and transferred care to the medical team that had gathered. I gave the story and stood back, watching them work.

Five minutes passed. More epi, atropine, then sodium bicarb. I gave up hope. The room was a flurry of activity, noisy, a little chaotic. I saw the boy's parents outside the door, the mom now crying, stunned, the father now in shock.

"We've got a pulse."

"The room went still. Sure enough a rhythm appeared on the monitor, sinus tach. A few minutes later I saw my patient open his eyes and look around the room.

It's kind of strange what happened next. I was fully prepared for him to die. Whatever it is we have inside us making it possible to do this job was in full operation. I didn't feel anything, not sadness, despair, or frustration. I knew we did our job, and the outcome was out of our hands. I was at peace with that.

Whatever it is that allows us to do this job disappeared as soon as I heard he had a pulse. When I saw him open his eyes my own eyes filled with tears. It was strange, but I'll take it over emptiness any day.

It's good to know I still have a heart.

Reprinted with permission from EMS World

Wounded

The early morning sun had yet to break the horizon as we approached the two-family home in the heart of South Providence. Places like this are everywhere in the neighborhoods, well-kept multifamily homes, some a little dated, others freshly painted with ornate metal gates adorning the driveways. There was no gate here, just an old Ford parked next to the house, with a wounded combat veteran license plate on the back.

A trend has resurfaced in this neighborhood. Somebody buys a two- or three-family home, Mom and Pop live on the ground floor, the kids who own the place occupy the second, and, if available, the third apartment is rented, sometimes to another family member, to help foot the bill. My own family started out like this; it actually sounds kind of nice. Absentee landlords still exploit the poor folks who settle here, their homes obviously lacking the TLC needed to maintain the old places.

I walked into the home. The old folks lived on the first floor. It looked like they had lived there for decades. Slumped in a kitchen chair was our patient, an eighty-five-year-old veteran named Joe. Engine 11 had arrived first, an IV was already established, vital signs taken and high-flow oxygen being delivered through a non-rebreather. Joe had tried to take a sip of his morning coffee, felt sudden weakness, and spilled it all over his crisp, white T-shirt. There was obvious facial droop, and no strength on his left side when he squeezed my hands.

His wife of fifty years stood by, nervously wiping the spilled coffee from the green linoleum floor. "He goes to the VA," she said.

As the guys from the 11 and Adam helped Joe into the stair chair, having to strap him tight so he wouldn't tip to the left, I took his wife to the side. I hated doing it.

"When did you notice something different?" I asked.

"Right before I called you, about ten minutes ago. He was fine, drinking his coffee like he does every day, then he dropped it and couldn't tell me what was wrong."

"I think Joe is having a stroke," I said as gently and quickly as I could. "If we get him to the proper facility the damage can be stopped. We can help him but the VA isn't the best place for something like this."

She started to argue, insurance reasons maybe, familiarity more likely, but saw the urgency in my gaze and relented.

"I'll stay here and clean up," she replied, nervously wiping the kitchen table where the coffee-stained paper sat, opened to the sports section.

In the truck Joe was in the stretcher, listing to the left.

"Let's go."

I reassessed his vital signs and tried to get him to speak. He tried valiantly but was frustrated and unable to articulate his thoughts.

As we sped to the ER, I gave him the news. A wounded World War II vet deserved the truth.

"Joe, you are having a stroke. There are treatments available and we're within the time frame. We can stop the damage; you're not done fighting just yet."

His right hand gripped mine fiercely, he made eye contact, then he closed his eyes. We rode to the hospital in silence, him lost in his thoughts, me hoping I wasn't witnessing his last battle.

Reprinted with permission from Fire Engineering

Just Once

"Rescue 1, respond with Ladder 5 to 990 Broad Street, at the pay phone for a fifty-year-old female experiencing chest pain."

"Rescue 1, responding."

Housework had been underway when the tone hit. Me and Rob dropped our mops and made for the apparatus floor. A miniature dust cloud swept through the garage as the overhead door opened, inviting the cold wind into our home. The remains of a late-winter snowstorm lingered on the roads of Providence where salt and sand accumulated, then stuck to our trucks as we plowed through the slush. When the ice melts from the vehicles a deposit is made on the floor, and we spread it around as we walk to and from the vehicles. The floor is swept daily; we just can't keep up. Spring cleaning is around the corner, that and warmer weather should clean things up.

Chest pain at the pay phone at 990 Broad Street at eight in the morning. Ninety-nine times out of one hundred this is a call for somebody who had been smoking crack all night. It is difficult to not get tunnel vision but I try to stay objective.

"Ladder 5 to fire alarm, advise rescue we have a fifty-year-old female, chest pain radiating down her left arm, diaphoretic, obtaining vitals."

"Rescue 1, received." This patient sounded like the one out of a hundred.

Ladder 5's crew had obtained vital signs, administered aspirin and oxygen, and had a nitro on board when we arrived on scene. The woman looked like she just left a PTA meeting in one of the suburbs surrounding Providence. We loaded her into the rescue and continued care, first running an EKG, then starting a line. Vitals signs weren't great, 160/100 after a nitro with a pulse of 120. The EKG read sinus tach. The patient looked anxious but her skin was now cool and dry.

Ladder 5 went back in service after doing most of my work; Rob and I transported the patient to the ER at Rhode Island Hospital. En route I found that the patient had been out all night looking for her car, which had been "stolen" by an acquaintance. I didn't want to ask, but had to.

"Did you do any drugs last night?"

"I had to smoke some to keep awake."

"Smoke what?"

"Crack."

One hundred out of one hundred.

Retraining

We're just people. Sure, we're trained in advanced lifesaving techniques; yes we have at our disposal tools to be used in lifesaving efforts. We have experience, know-how, and that special something that keeps us sane when time and time again all we do isn't enough.

We get called when all else has failed. The finality of death is overwhelming when it comes unexpectedly. Most people watch, wishing they knew what to do but paralyzed by fear. There is no room for second-guessing when a person has stopped breathing. Decisions must be made without thinking; actions carried out automatically, procedures followed, and work to be done.

When all we do isn't enough, when a person dies before his time, all we have is the knowledge that we did all we could. Sometimes it is all we have.

Two off-duty nurses took it upon themselves to call the head of Emergency Medical Services in Providence to express their dissatisfaction with two of our best EMTs during an incident last week. A man in his fifties died in a restaurant. Our people did everything in their power to save the man's life, and took it hard when all they had wasn't enough. The head of Emergency Medical Services placated the nurses, told them he would send the EMTs in question for retraining.

I think they learned enough that night.

Thank God we have each other.

Different Views

He lay facedown in the street, a stab wound to the back of his head and a bleeding lump on his forehead. A butcher knife reflected the streetlight's glow three feet from his head and a broken golf club rested near his feet.

He was conscious, barely. We put some gauze on front and back of his head to stop the bleeding, put him in a c-collar, rolled him onto a spine board, and put him in back of the rescue. As we started an IV and did a secondary assessment, a police officer stuck his head into the back of the rescue.

"Has he been drinking?" he asked.

"Looks like it," I replied.

"Maybe he tripped and fell," suggested the cop.

"Maybe he got stabbed in the back of the head with a butcher knife and clubbed on the forehead with a nine iron," I replied.

It's all in how you look at things, and more importantly, how you report them.

Violent crime is down in Providence for the fourth straight year.

Relapse

He walked into the Dunkin' Donuts in Olneyville, asked the help to call 911, then collapsed into the puddle his dripping clothing created. He said no more until we arrived.

"I got hit in the head with something hard," he explained. "Then they threw me into the river."

I did a primary evaluation and didn't see any sign of trauma, no bleeding, no deformities, bumps, or bruises. He told me he had a history of substance abuse but had been clean for months.

"Can you call my mother?" he asked.

We put him into the rescue, stripped off his soaked clothing, and wrapped him in blankets. I took off my coat and cranked up the heat. He gave me his mother's number and I dialed. She answered on the first ring, sounding exhausted.

"Hello, this is Lieutenant Morse with the Providence Fire Department. I have your son in the ambulance; he's not injured but appears to have been out all night. We're taking him to Rhode Island Hospital for an evaluation."

I handed the phone to our patient; he talked for a minute, then was quiet.

We got him to the hospital and transferred care in a few minutes. As I left the ER, a middle-aged couple and girl about the patient's age walked over to me.

"Excuse me, are you the Providence firefighter who called from the rescue?"

They looked to me for answers concerning their family member's ordeal. I honestly couldn't tell them much more than I already had—he was out all night, says he was assaulted and ended up on a riverbank in Olneyville.

He had been paid that morning and planned to visit his kids in another state by way of Kennedy Plaza, the city's bus station. It also serves as the city's place to get in all kinds of trouble with all kinds of people and all kinds of substances.

The family is holding out hope that he was mugged. I wish I shared their faith in his sobriety.

Smoking Kills

He stood outside the apartment with his girlfriend, waiting for the ambulance. His skin was grey when we arrived, the front of his shirt soaked with blood. We got him into the truck, cut off his clothes, put him on oxygen, started two lines, and ran an EKG. His vitals were crashing, 90/62, HR 120, SpO2 90% on 10 liters. Engine Co. 6 from Hartford Ave. assisted, Heidi helped in back, the captain drove the rescue, and Coley followed with the engine. We have been through similar jobs, everything went like clockwork.

He was stabbed in the chest by his friend. They were in the friend's apartment watching TV. Our patient, now in critical condition in the Rhode Island Hospital trauma intensive care unit, lit up a smoke. His friend told him not to smoke in the apartment. Our patient puffed away. His friend rendered his lungs incapable of inhaling, one of them anyway, pneumothorax, right lung.

I stayed in the trauma room for a while, watching the ER doctors decompress the pleural space. A doctor felt inside the hole for any tearing of the diaphragm. Then they stuck a chest tube between the ribs and relieved the pressure that had built there. Buckets of blood poured from the tube onto the stretcher as the patient screamed in pain.

It looks like he will survive the ordeal. When we were kids, me and my brother loved nothing more than watching the *Creature Double Feature* on an old TV in our basement on Saturday afternoons, occasionally erupting into a battle royale on the basement floor before the second part of the double feature began.

This was quite a different kind of Saturday afternoon matinee.

Complacency Kills

Monday she was drunk at home, a concerned friend called 911 to have strangers check on her well-being. I guess it is easier to call the fire department when a friend is in need than getting up and doing something yourself. We found her inside her apartment, empty beer cans littering the floor, highly intoxicated. There is no law against being drunk at home but our patient clearly needed some help. After a small brawl we talked her into going to the hospital for detox, hopefully eventual rehab.

Wednesday she was home again, drunk. This time she called 911 for a ride to the hospital because she wanted to go to detox. Apparently, rehab wasn't in the cards on Monday.

Saturday we got a call for an intoxicated person at an address on Broad Street. It was our friend, drunk again, this time at an acquaintance's place. He was tired of her, wanted us to get rid of his "problem." By now I thought we had become friends. It's a short trip to the emergency room, but a bond quickly forms between patient and caregiver, especially a "frequent flyer."

Monday we got a call for a person down in the bushes. I saw a hand rise from some hedges in front of one of the high-rises that the elderly and disabled residents of Providence reside in. Walking closer I saw my old friend, drunk again, unable to extricate herself from where she fell. She fought for a while, learned quickly that one fifty-six-year-old former prostitute is no match for five firefighters sent to help her. "I have a knife," she said, enraged now that we had her out of her nest.

You would think that after all these years I would learn never to let my guard down. Because familiarity sets in by no means diminishes the potential threat on every call. To the patients we are sent to treat we are no more than a blur, a momentary diversion from their otherwise dreary existence. Once we part ways we are forgotten, the next person who enters their lives more important than the last.

She ripped open the front of her coat and brandished a twelve-inch butcher's knife. Her eyes were wild, full of hate. Before she had a chance to hurt herself, or us, we disarmed her, put her on the stretcher, and took her to the hospital. There was no real malice once the knife was out of her hands, but for one moment, when she was capable of murder, she could have altered a lot of lives.

Pink Hippopotamuses
Our patient lay on her back in an oversized bed, covered with blankets. Just her face peeped out from under the covers.

"What is the matter?" I asked.

"I feel like I've been drugged."

"How does that feel?"

"I'm all woozy and happy."

"Did you take any drugs?"

"Just some Oxycontin."

"When did you take the Oxycontin?"

"Right before I started feeling like I was drugged."

Hippopotamus one, hippopotamus two, hippopotamus three . . .

She had a prescription for Oxycontin to help with some pain she had been experiencing following the birth a week ago of her daughter. Her family gathered around the bed as I explained that the effects she was feeling were perfectly normal and to be expected after taking a painkiller.

"That is exactly what the doctor said," the baby's father offered from the foot of the bed. "We just wanted to make sure so we called 911."

I swear I don't make these things up.

Stretcher?
Fuel?
    Check.
Lights and siren?
    Check.
Medications, IV equipment?
    Check, check.

Splints, bandages, and peroxide?
Check, check, check!
Stretcher?
Stretcher?
Stretcher?
Just when you think you are a hero, somebody from East Providence needs an ambulance and you don't have a stretcher. Too bad we didn't realize it before we got there. Thankfully, firefighters are a kind, forgiving lot and understand a little mistake. I'm sure this little faux pas will be forgotten quickly.

That and I've got a bridge for sale in Brooklyn.

Let Me Out!

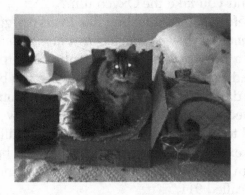

I was wondering what happened to Victoria, she had been missing since we moved. Poor thing had to chew her way out of the box we packed her in!

Nailed

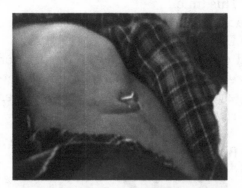

Every now and then the wrong thing gets nailed.

Here We Go Again

I just transported a psychiatric patient from Butler Hospital to Miriam Hospital, a trip of about three miles. The patient was in Butler for a variety of reasons; today we were called for her medical problem. We were escorted through the hospital grounds by a security guard who led us to the ambulance bay. From there, another security guard walked us to the unit where our patient waited. Security was tight; we were escorted through a locked door into the patient area. Our patient was stable; we put her onto our stretcher and asked if security would be coming with us. "No," was the answer. "We do this all the time, no security necessary."

I could, and maybe should have made an issue out of the situation but felt as though I would be pushing water uphill. We left the facility, escorted by security until we left the hospital grounds. From there we were on our own. While reading the patients report it was noted in multiple places that the patient was volatile, unpredictable, and prone to violence. Among other things she tried to kill her mother and sister. The psych evaluation was a day old. The trip was uneventful. This time.

Security at Miriam Hospital will keep an eye on her while she is treated.

This kind of thing goes on every day, nationwide. EMS providers are left vulnerable. Going along to get along will eventually get, and probably already has gotten somebody seriously hurt, or killed.

Providence Burning

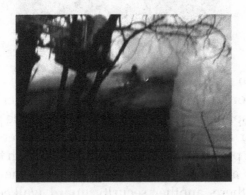

There are over a thousand vacant, boarded-up houses in Providence. The three major fires we fought today were in occupied buildings. Four or five others, small fires, we put out before they could get going, one in the basement of a day care. Two firefighters suffered injuries that required an emergency room visit; many more were able to walk their injuries off and keep fighting.

Night has arrived. Vacant houses have a tendency to ignite when the sun goes down.

Stay safe, brothers and sisters, the night is young.

A Few Seconds

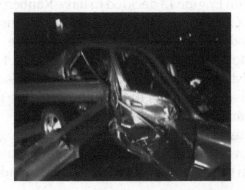

What a difference a few seconds makes. Two young women were travelling home at about four this morning when their car lost control, straddled the highway divider, took out a hundred feet of guardrail, and ended up facing the wrong way on the other side of Route 195. But for a few mph more, a twist or turn in either direction, or the tiniest flick of the steering wheel during the crash, the guardrail would have intruded the front passenger compartment rather than the empty backseat.

The girls walked away with minor injuries. Their families and friends now have the opportunity to see them grow older, pursue their lives, maybe someday start a family of their own. The girls themselves, having never seen the mangled bodies that have littered these highways over the years, will probably never know just how lucky they are to be alive. Those of us who have seen the dead and dying know, and are thankful that these two didn't join all the others that left heartbroken families and friends where the miracle of life, hope, and future generations should have been.

Where's the Rye?

The guys from Engine 13 decided to have Reuben sandwiches for lunch. Corned beef, Swiss cheese, Thousand Island dressing, and a little sauerkraut grilled on rye. Great idea. They went to a local market, got the corned beef, Swiss, and Thousand Island but couldn't get the rest. Rescue 1 to the rescue! We have the run of the city and can go to more stores. "No problem," I said and started my quest.

Three runs and five stores later, with nothing but an old can of yellow sauerkraut I found on the bottom shelf of a Spanish market to show for my troubles, I made it back to the station.

Rye bread?

I had a better chance of finding Osama bin Laden in Providence. What the heck is going on around here?

The New Rescue 1

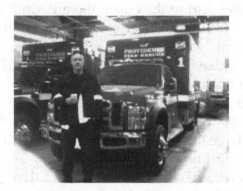

Coming soon to a street near you, the new, improved Rescue 1.

Too bad it's the same old crew. Fifty-five-year-old guy dead in the rescue, CPR, asystolic, didn't get a line until we were at the hospital, couldn't intubate, didn't see the piece of hot dog stuck in his throat, time of death 1635 hrs.

Saved another heroin addict at 1400 hrs. A guy in his forties, dead on the floor of his kitchen. A friend found him just in time. 2 mg Narcan to the rescue. I wish there were an antidote to choking.

Line of the Week

The ER was a madhouse, drunken street people, drunken college kids, drunken housewives, drunken fools. Minor injuries, a few legitimate traumas, some sick old folks and a bunch of people vomiting. The wait was hours. In the middle of it all was a twenty-something-year-old inmate from the ACI and two correctional officers. The prisoner had a minor injury to his throat from an altercation and had been waiting for a long time. As I walked past them I overheard the inmate ask his guards, "Can I go back to my cell? Anywhere is better than here."

Who's the Guy?

"This isn't funny anymore," he said as he stumbled toward the rescue.

"I never thought it was."

"I'm tired."

"You're a mess."

He sat on the bench seat, five feet away from me, not far enough to keep the stale piss mixed with fresh vodka smell from invading my space. Truth be told, it doesn't bother me anymore, just a minor annoyance to be tolerated during the short ride to the ER. He is fifty-two, close to the end of his run. I have seen a lot of people like him die on the streets in their early fifties. I think he knows.

"You're running out of time," I told him. He looked back at me and gave me a lopsided grin.

"Who's the guy, that was a famous race car driver, but crashed against a wall, and died."

"I thought this wasn't fun anymore."

He cocked an eyebrow and stared at me.

"Number 3, Dale Earhart."

"You are correct!"

"Who's the guy, that played Ben Hur, and just died?" I asked.

"You're asking the questions?"

"Might as well."

He didn't know the answer.

Babysitters

A young man sat swaying on the steps in front of a house on Orms Street. Rob pulled the rescue to a stop in front of him. I stepped out of the truck and a middle-aged woman handed me a cell phone.

"Hello," I said.

"My brother has been drinking and has to go to the hospital," was the message from the other side. If I were anywhere but Providence I would have thought I had entered the twilight zone.

"Really," I said. The last three calls were starting to get to me. People are becoming more brazen in their abuse of the 911 system. An "emotional" female who had broken up with her boyfriend called 911 because she was upset, a fifteen-year-old girl tasted some nail polish remover because some kids at school said she would get high, another fifteen-year-old girl sat in her family's car as her parents waited for an ambulance to take her to Hasbro Children's Hospital because her cramps were extra bad. The hospital was two blocks away; I could see the entrance ramp from their driveway. They wanted to get right in.

"Who is this?" I asked.

"It don't matter, just get him to the hospital," came the reply.

"You just try taking me to the hospital, there's gonna be trouble," from the guy sitting on the steps.

At this point I should have called for the police and left the scene but my curiosity got the best of me. That and I knew they would just call us back to transport an intoxicated male.

"Where are you calling from?" I asked the caller.

"Coventry." Coventry is a suburb of Providence, fifteen minutes away.

"Then get in your car and take care of your brother yourself," I said.

"I can't. I don't feel good."

A guy who I assumed to be the young man's father stumbled out of the house and stood staring at us.

"Either take care of your problem or the police are coming," I said. He said nothing, the drunk guy continued to sway.

"Is this your son?" I asked the woman who had handed me the phone. She stared at me as well.

"Do you speak English?" I asked everybody. Nothing. The drunk guy was the only person I could communicate with.

Defeated, I helped the drunk guy to his feet and told him we were going to the hospital and there wasn't going to be any trouble. He believed me and stayed quiet during the thirty-second transport to Roger Williams Medical Center. The man on the porch slurred something in English and walked back inside with the woman, their problem solved by the Providence Fire Department.

I don't know how it happened, but we have become society's babysitters.

Gang's All Here
Joe and Harold, Kevin and Jimmy, I got those four.

Stephan and Beetlejuice came by way of Rescue 5.

Rescue 3 is going downtown for a female, intoxicated.

Al and Ronny will be in Rescue 2 any minute.

The CDU (Clinical Decision Unit) at Rhode Island Hospital is filling up fast. It's early yet; where will all the drunk people go?

What's Worse?

"Rescue 1 and Engine 11, respond to I-95 in the center travel lane for a motorcycle accident."

"Rescue 1 on the way."

"Tony, take a left on Eddy Street, we'll take a look from the overpass."

"That can't be good," said Tony as we approached. Four or five cars had stopped on the bridge and were looking below onto the highway.

"Traffic's backed up," I said, noticing the line of cars on the highway that had backed up as far as I could see.

"There he is," said Tony, pointing to a figure lying in the road, a motorcycle about fifty feet in front of him on its side.

"Take the Thurber's on-ramp north, we'll back up to the incident," I said.

Tony took the ramp and we entered the highway. Cars sped past us. We had gone too far and were now a hundred yards in front of the victim.

"Shit, I thought the traffic would be stopped. Go to the next exit we'll have to circle around."

Tony gunned it. The next exit was a mile up the road; we would have to take that one, travel south for about two miles, turn around again, then approach the accident from the south.

"I shouldn't have tried that," I said. Minutes can make all the difference and I just blew about five.

"It should have worked," said Tony. "You would think the traffic would have at least slowed."

"Engine 11 to fire alarm, on scene."

Tony had turned the rescue around; we were flying down the highway trying to make up some time. I couldn't help think that if this guy died it was on me.

"Engine 11 to fire alarm, advise Rescue 1 we have a twenty-three-year-old female complaining of a headache, alert and conscious, no trauma."

"Rescue 1 received," I said into the mic, leaned back in my seat, and breathed normally for the first time in four minutes. A minute later we arrived on scene. Our patient was shaken up, lost some skin on her right side and ruined the paint job on her helmet. It was a full-face kind and probably saved her life, if not permanent disfigurement. She was "going about seventy," felt the bike wobble and remembered nothing else until another motorist shook her and asked if she was all right. The entire surface of the helmet was badly damaged, hard plastic that would have been her skin and hair if she had chosen to go without.

We put her on the spine board and collar, put her in the truck, and took her to the trauma room at Rhode Island Hospital. She nearly fainted when I started an IV.

"I hate needles!" she cried when I punctured her skin, moaning in pain. She hadn't made a peep until now.

"You just crashed a motorcycle at seventy miles an hour and you're crying about a little needle?"

"Yeah, but this is different!"

I understood. I hate needles too. I pushed the catheter home.

Seizure

She sat on the floor in the office of the soup kitchen, semiconscious.

"What happened?" I asked the lady in charge.

"She had a seizure."

"Can you describe the seizure?"

"She was shaking."

"Let's go, Ella," I said to the lady sitting on the floor. She looked up at me, gave a half smile, and slowly got to her feet. I picked up her belongings, a basket-weave beach bag filled with clothing and other personal things. On top was a pair of new Keds.

"They gave me new sneakers," Ella said as we walked toward the rescue. "Make sure you don't lose them."

"You didn't have a seizure, did you?" I asked, once we were alone.

"No. I just don't belong out here. I can't do it. I'm scared."

"Where were you before this?"

"Butler Hospital. I was there for six months. Once they were done with the shock treatments they had to let me go."

"Did the shocks help?"

"Yeah, but I'm not ready to be out here. I don't like it."

"Do you have any family?"

"Thirty-two grandchildren," she said proudly.

"No wonder you were in a psychiatric facility," I said.

"They visit once a week. It takes me three days to clean up after them."

We arrived at the hospital. As we wheeled her in she started shaking.

Maybe they'll keep her.

Thanks

They had a nice time visiting the zoo at Roger Williams Park; the kids were tired but satisfied after a day of fun. The baby, sixteen months old, seemed a little more tired than his three-year-old sister. The mom and dad got concerned when they couldn't wake him up. They called 911 and waited in their minivan for help to arrive. The little guy was still unconscious when we arrived. He moved his foot a little when his mom tickled him.

"Has he ever had a seizure?" I asked.

"Febrile seizures about six months ago but he's been fine since."

Rob took his temperature, 102.4. Maybe it was another seizure.

"Did you witness any seizure activity?" I asked.

"He didn't shake but he did look a little dazed when we put him in the van, then this."

I can't even imagine how awful the parents must have felt at that point. They travelled about an hour from Massachusetts for a nice family day. They had no idea where the hospital was or how to find it. Providence is a tricky place, there are a lot of unsavory places one can get lost in while looking for help.

Rob assessed the blood pressure and SpO2 and I checked the baby's BG level, started him on oxygen and got rolling, planning to attempt an IV en route. I explained to the family that febrile seizures are common, what their child was experiencing I had seen hundreds of times.

One of the best parts of my job is having the opportunity to come into people's lives, albeit briefly, and make an impact that will stay with them for a long, long time. The parents were frantic, the three-year-old frightened and crying, and the baby unresponsive. Within two minutes of our arrival the baby and mom were in the back of Rescue 1, calm and confidant everything would be okay, the dad and his daughter on their way to the ER, following the foolproof directions Lieutenant Grantham from Engine 11 gave them.

The baby had regained consciousness when we backed into Hasbro Children's Hospital. I passed on the information we had documented to Nancy, the RN in charge of triage. On the way out the dad stopped me, shook my hand, and said, "Thanks."

Hamada

Strange how things happen. It was four in the morning; Rescue 1 was unavailable, dead battery. While waiting for the mechanic from the repair shop to arrive and get us going I randomly searched VerveEarth for blogs from around the world, eventually landing in the UK and Susie Hemingway's site, http://www.susiehemingway.blogspot. com. Something compelled me to hang around. This poem hit home in so many ways. Heroes are all around us, fighting life-and-death battles, facing the fear of uncertainty and the unknown yet still are able to inspire others during the darkest days of their lives. People previously unknown to me and living on another continent are fighting cancer with amazing grace, dignity, and courage.

Keep fighting, Hamada and Susie, but just as important: keep living!

>*"We Dance Again"*
>*No wretched life from us can take*
>*the steps of love the notes we make,*
>*the frail frame that yearns to try*
>*the arms that lift, the eyes that cry,*
>*tiny steps are all you need*
>*to close your eyes and dance with me*
>*to swirl and sway, to waltz and salsa*
>*maybe soon – but not today,*
>*still just to hold and smell your skin*
>*is all I need, not spin and twirl*
>*your arms are weak your legs move slow*
>*but in this room the music flows*
>*do you hear Count Basie swing?*
>*piano notes that damp your skin*
>*just as snow when flakes begin*
>*to see you there upon this floor*

to hear that sax in blues begin
to twirl and spin,
close your eyes and drift again
tiny steps are all you'll need
to turn on floor, so close to me
for I will hold you never fear
and as we dance along this year
tiny steps are all you need
so close your eyes and dance with me . . .

Susie Hemingway

Refugee

He's twelve years old, been in this country for three years. He was crossing the busy part of Elmwood Avenue, right in front of the library at dusk, when either he walked into a moving auto or the moving auto hit him. The stories from the driver and the pedestrian are never the same. The only thing I really cared about was the patent's injuries. He held his right foot in the cradle of his hands. I sat next to him on the sidewalk and asked him where he was hurt.

"Just my ankle," he said, solemn, his eyes never making contact with my own, his head bent toward the ground. I noticed scars on his head, long healed but still prominent through neatly cropped hair. His father was at home, a few streets over. I got a phone for him to use from Ariel, one of the firefighters from Engine 11 who had been called to assist with a child struck by an auto.

Abdi pushed the right buttons but nobody answered. We helped him to the back of the rescue, where Rob took his vital signs. Abdi pushed up his sleeve to make room for the blood pressure cuff and exposed an eight-inch scar running the length of his arm. Rob and I saw the scar, looked at each other, then at Abdi, who looked away.

He didn't say much, didn't smile or relax the way most boys eventually do when with Providence firefighters. He answered our questions politely and let us put ice on his ankle. On the way to the hospital I asked where he came from.

"Africa," he replied.

"Is it nice there?" I asked, knowing the street where he lived to be one of the worst in Providence. Abdi looked afraid and shook his head quickly from side to side. "Where in Africa?" I asked.

"Somalia." He mumbled the word, almost like it was a curse. I sat back on the bench seat and wondered what kind of life this poor kid led before escaping to this country. And what kind of life lay ahead of him.

Wounds

He wasn't concerned about his face; he was more concerned with revenge. Two guys "snaked" him, snuck up behind him and slashed him with knives. The right side of his face wasn't too bad, a two-inch laceration, not too deep. The left side was wide open, from his ear to his chin; I could see his jawbone. Another slice went from his nose to the corner of his mouth. The back of his neck sported another gash.

When the police asked him if he wanted to press charges, he said he didn't know his attackers.

"You are going to be scarred for life," I told him. He wasn't impressed. "A fraction of an inch lower and you would have bled to death before we got here." He didn't believe me. "Those guys tried to kill you," I told him.

"No shit, Pop," he said nonchalantly. "And I'm going to kill them."

This morning he was a handsome nineteen-year-old kid, charismatic in an inner city kind of way, with his life ahead of him. Today at 1600 hrs. all of that changed. Now his face and his soul are scarred, and his future uncertain.

Extreme Makeover

Sometimes it's good to take a time-out and enjoy the good things life has to offer. Last night was one of those nights. A few pizzas, a couple of dips with some nachos, sodas, beer, wine, and my family sitting in my new family room watching ABC's *Extreme Makeover*, Rhode Island edition. It seems some TV executive finally got it right; instead of spending millions of dollars creating and producing mindless drivel that does nothing but fritter time away from a bored audience, Ty Pennington and crew find people in need of a break, get the community involved, muster up as much positive energy they can, and make the world a better place, not only for the deserving people who are the center of all the attention, but everybody who helped as well. And don't forget the audience: I sat with my wife, Cheryl, plus Danielle, Brittany, and Eric for an hour watching the show and loved every second of it. The house that they built is a mile away from my own or I probably never would have known about this show.

I have an EMT student riding the rescue today. Turns out his day job is a CVS Samaritan, one of the guys that ride the highway at rush hour helping motorists in need of a fixed flat tire, gasoline, or whatever else to get them going or get off the highway to a safe place. He says he loves his job. I think he's kind of like a mini version of the *Extreme Makeover* crew, only on the highway. Come to think of it, I'm kind of like the *Extreme Makeover* crew, only in an ambulance.

Tuesday Morning Madness

Tuesday morning and things are off to a great start. At 0700 hrs. a forty-six-year-old guy had his wife drive him to the ER at RIH because of chest pains. They made it to the parking lot and couldn't get any farther. We were called and found a diaphoretic patient in obvious distress. We got an IV going, put him on oxygen, aspirin, and nitro, ran an EKG, and brought him in. Turns out he was having an anterior wall MI. Thirty minutes later he was in the cath lab, where they opened his blocked artery.

0830, a twenty-six-year-old mother of two was approached on Messer Street by a woman looking to buy some crack. The mother of two was familiar with the drug seeker but had never spoken to her. She tried to get away, the drug seeker went into a frenzy and stabbed and sliced the mother. She's in the trauma room at Rhode Island Hospital, lacerations to her face and arms and a stab wound to her abdomen. Strange day so far.

Dumbfellas
A couple of nineteen-year-olds thought it would be a good idea to come to South Providence and settle a score with somebody. They put on their wife-beaters, shined up their gold jewelry, slicked back their hair, and rode into town looking to bust some heads. I think the theme from *The Sopranos* was playing when they rolled in. A little while later I drove them out of the hood in the ambulance, bloodied and bruised, minus their car. They were lucky to get out alive.

"People came from everywhere," they told me. "There must have been thirty of them."

I guess they haven't been watching the news. Every night there have been multiple stabbings and shots fired.

Kids from the suburbs think they know what goes on in the inner city. They play the part of tough guys, believe that they are, and get themselves into all kinds of trouble when they find out that what they think they know, just isn't so.

DOA

He died last night, fell off the side of his bed, tipped a lamp over and died on the floor. He was an old man, from the looks of things lived a simple life. His possessions were few, modest furniture, not a lot of clothes, just the necessities. We stood there after pronouncing him dead and waited for the police sergeant, five of us, strangers to the dead man, talking about our weekend, our kids, our future.

His grandson arrived, walked past us and kneeled by his grandfather's side, sobbing.

Another grandson ran into the room and joined them next to the bed. The phone rang; another family member entered the room. The police arrived, we backed out. As we were leaving I saw another young man running toward the house, frantic.

He may not have had many worldly possessions, but from the look of the people he left behind, he knew how to live.

Out with the Old, In with the . . . Old

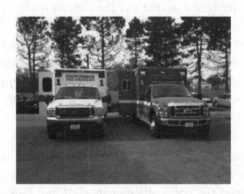

We finally put the new red truck in service yesterday. There was a big party, steamship round, open bar, Billy Joel did a tribute to the men and women of Rescue 1, and to top it off, Angelina Jolie, dressed in a stunning Armani, christened the new truck by smashing a bottle of Dom Pérignon right before we embarked on our first run.

The "new car" scent lasted ten minutes, quickly replaced by the "old rescue" odor of one of our regulars. He called from a pay phone half a mile from Rhode Island Hospital, said he was "sick." The smell of piss, alcohol, and vomit, mixed with a month's worth of filth, quickly filled our new environment. Oh well.

Lieutenant Pagano

I worked with Lt. James Pagano's father for a few years, back in the eighties. I didn't know Lieutenant Pagano, but if he was anything like his father, we have lost a true gentleman. Rest in peace, Brother Pagano, my condolences to the family.

Providence Journal

May 22, 2008

For slain firefighter, a line out the door at wake

CRANSTON — They began lining up around 3 this afternoon outside the funeral home to say goodbye to slain Cranston firefighter Lt. James A. Pagano — firefighters in dress blues and white gloves and solemn faces, friends and family.

Firefighters from Cranston, Providence, Bristol, Coventry and elsewhere have come to pay respects at the wake for Pagano, who the police allege was shot and killed Sunday by next-door neighbor Nicholas Gianquitti, 40. Gianquitti, a former Providence police officer, is now charged with murder.

Pagano "was a great guy, the ultimate family guy," said James Moore, who retired as a Cranston deputy fire chief in 2002 and worked with Pagano at Station 3 for several years.

At first there were two lines to get into Nardolillo Funeral Home, with firefighters in one and friends and family in another. Shortly before 5 p.m., about 100 people were waiting to go inside.

The full Cranston command staff and the chief are inside with Pagano's family.

An American flag flew at half-staff.

Bookworthy
I take a lot of good-natured ribbing from the guys on the job, they ask me during runs if this is "bookworthy," or "did I make the book?" I honestly have no idea why some things make it here and others don't. I do make an attempt to not sensationalize other people's tragedies; a lot of the more dramatic things that go on never make it here. Just for kicks, whatever happens next is officially "bookworthy." Stay tuned . . .

Not Bookworthy
1050 hrs. Rescue 2 (overtime) responds to a one-family home in the west end for a ninety-two-year-old female having trouble breathing. Visiting nurse on scene states patient's pulsox is 40. Impossible you say? So did I.

Arrived on scene to find ninety-two-year-old female in bathroom with the door closed. The visiting nurse informed us that the patient walked in to relieve herself before going to the hospital. "Is she breathing?" I asked. The nurse opened the door and said, "Yes."

We took her to the hospital; I never did put her on our pulsox machine. The patient looked fine and stated she was having no difficulty breathing. Machines can't always be depended on; you have to trust the patient sometimes.

In my opinion, this post is definitely not bookworthy, but then, it is a good example of a lot of our calls.

Sunrise

Another sunrise. For some, anyway. A Cranston firefighter lays in his grave, buried yesterday after being shot in the back by his neighbor. While his family grieves, sleepless in their home, another man is shot in the back on Atwells Avenue, a few miles away. He has bullets in both of his legs and a hole in his back but is still alive, conscious, and in the trauma room at Rhode Island Hospital. My guess is he wasn't delivering newspapers when he was gunned down at dawn. Maybe he was an innocent victim, wrong place, wrong time. Probably not. He's alive, the firefighter is not. The senselessness of it all is overwhelming.

I'm finishing thirty-eight, can't wait to get home, an hour to go.

Rock Stars

I wondered what all the limos were doing downtown; rows of them lined up near the Westin, in front of the Biltmore, and parked around Kennedy Plaza. I thought some dignitaries from an oil-rich Arab country were in town or something similar. These weren't "economy" limousines, they were brand new, bright white Cadillacs, Lincolns, Hummers— somebody even had a stretch pickup truck. There were dozens of them. Turns out a high school was holding their senior prom at a downtown hotel.

Later, we responded to a popular nightclub for a possible overdose. An eighteen-year-old girl was found lying on her back in an alley next to the club, her tiny black dress covered with vomit. Her friends were concerned. They had graduated from a private high school that afternoon and were out celebrating. Hundreds of bleary-eyed kids swarmed the rescue, taking pictures with their camera phones, laughing, shouting, partying full speed ahead. I asked the friends what happened, they said they didn't know. The unconscious girl was in the VIP room at the club and ended up in the alley. We got her to the ER where she threw up again, this time on one of the ER technicians.

I wonder if the idea of a prom in the high school gym and a graduation party in the backyard ever occurred to these folks. Life isn't always glamorous. Truly special occasions lose their luster when every little milestone is celebrated as if it were a glorious achievement. A little humility early in life leaves something to look forward to later on. Everybody wants to be a rock star, most of us won't be.

Jumper

It was his fourth attempt that I'm aware of, two by hanging, one by a wrist slashing. This time he jumped thirty feet from a highway overpass onto the pavement. Rescue 1 was dispatched as a special signal and directed to respond to the highway below the overpass using a silent approach. The highway was jammed; traffic had been stopped on both sides for ten minutes before we were dispatched. Stephanie, my chauffeur for the evening, got us as close as possible before things got too tight to move forward. Rather than use the sirens we waited about a quarter-mile away from the incident and hoped for the best. After ten minutes the call came in from Ladder 1; the jumper had jumped. It took us a while to get to him; by the time we did the fire companies on scene had an IV established, cervical collar in place, and an EKG done. They had cut his clothes, exposing two fractured legs, a broken arm, broken ribs, and assorted scrapes and bruises. A carnival atmosphere had developed, crowds of people, some horrified but more than a few highly entertained by the spectacle.

We got him to the ER where last I heard he had no feeling in his legs. I guess he's lucky to be alive, but I'm really not sure if he thinks so.

So Am I

Eighty-two degrees, sunny skies, low humidity, perfect day. I refuse to let Providence's minions get me down, even though we're off to a shaky start.

0720 hrs. *"Rescue 1, respond to Veazie Street for a person with possible strep throat."*

911 for strep throat? Hmm. Could be an elderly person, high fever. Might be an infant. Could have breathing difficulties associated with the "possible strep throat." I kept an open mind during the response. The morning rush was on, traffic making the response twice as long. All Providence rescues are on other calls, Rescue 1 is sixth due to Veazie, on the "other" side of Providence. Lights and sirens all the way, some people go to great lengths to make room for the rescue, others are completely unaware of anything but themselves.

0732 hrs. "Rescue 1 on scene."

The apartment building is a disaster, kids' toys left haphazardly in the parking lot, trash bags ripped open by stray dogs, bottles broken, litter flying around, greasy finger marks smeared all over the doorbells. An empty coffee can held the door open a couple of inches, I kicked it in and walked up to the apartment. I knocked and waited. Knocked again and waited. Banged on the door with my radio. A thirtyish lady finally answered, bewildered expression on her face.

"Did you call for a rescue?"

"A rescue?"

"A rescue."

"I didn't call for no rescue."

"Somebody did."

"Hold on." She shut the door in my face. A few minutes later she came back.

"My son called from his room. You took him last night for a sore throat. I got to wait to get his medicine until eight o'clock but he's in pain."

"So am I."

Eighty-two degrees, sunny skies, low humidity, nearly perfect day. I probably won't let Providence's minions get to me.

Night and Day

Rhode Island Hospital ER, 0230 hrs.

Overdoses, stabbings, a man covered in blood and toothpaste (the blood was an offering to Jesus, the toothpaste protection from terrorists), drunks covered in vomit, people on backboards with cervical collars around their necks, a screaming man "four pointed" facedown on a stretcher, another guy trying to smash his head against the wall from his stretcher, a depressed man with stubs for feet sitting in a wheelchair crying, a sexual assault victim sobbing off to the side, sitting in the EMS break room talking to the police, and a little old lady who felt "faint" sitting in the middle of it all.

Alida, one of the two triage nurses, held it together with amazing grace but was about to lose it when the mother of a seventeen-year-old girl who had taken ten unknown pills demanded to be seen immediately and started acting up.

Things were about to hit the breaking point when two cars, followed by a trail of cops, sped into the ambulance bay and dumped a couple of gunshot victims onto the pavement. That quieted things down for a while as we got the victims onto stretchers and into the trauma rooms. My patient had a single GSW to his lower back, possibly shattering the lower spine. He was diaphoretic, hypotensive, and losing a lot of blood. The other victim ended up in another trauma room, a couple of bullet holes in him. I think the two were shooting at each other in a crowded nightclub parking lot.

I somehow got myself involved with the trauma team, along with Denny, a twenty-two-year-old "new guy" from Rescue 3. We started IVs, helped intubate, restrain, cut off clothes, and basically got bossed around by the trauma nurses and doctors. All hands on deck ruled the ER, too many patients, not enough hands.

An hour later we managed to extricate ourselves from the madness. Denny has been on rescue only two months but has already seen more than a lot of people will see for their entire career. If we can keep him humble we might let him stay in the rescue division.

Rhode Island Hospital ER, 0930 hrs.

New day, new hospital. The cops are gone, so are the maniacs. The trauma rooms are now full of elderly people, some with trouble breathing, others with chest pain, more with injuries from falls or MVAs. Last night's controlled chaos has been replaced with cool efficiency as tests are ordered, X-rays taken, and patients treated. The gunshot victims made it to the operating room, I think they will survive. What a difference a few hours makes.

Providence Journal

2 men shot outside Providence club

01:00 AM EDT on Sunday, June 15, 2008

PROVIDENCE – Two 22-year-old men were seriously injured yesterday in an early morning shooting and brawl outside a Poe Street club, the police said.

The two men were shot around 2 a.m. in the parking lot of the just-closed Platforms Dance Club. There are two clubs in the area, the police said.

There was a large disturbance in the parking lot and several shots rang out, said Sgt. James Marsland. It was a good-sized fight.

Injured were Derrick Knighton, of 139 Burnett St., Providence, and Derrick Clarke-Heath, address unknown. They were driven to Rhode Island Hospital by residents. Knighton was shot in the torso. Other patrons injured in the fight but not shot were also driven to the hospital for treatment, Marsland said.

Two patrolmen found .380-caliber shell casings in the parking lot. The police towed three cars believed to be involved in the fight: a 1994 Oldsmobile, a 1995 Chevy Lumina and a 1997 Nissan Maxima. No arrests have been made. The case is under investigation, Marsland said.

Little Angels

The cookout took a turn for the worse when a five-year-old girl fell down the stairs. Nothing life threatening but enough to put a damper on the festivities. She sat in her mother's arms crying softly when we arrived. A big bump and half-inch laceration decorated her forehead. Little kids just don't look right lying on a stretcher. Thankfully, my little patient was a perfect angel and might not even need a stitch. Her mother and two family members came with us to the hospital, the young girls translating for the mom. One of the girls told me she wants to write this summer, maybe become a novelist. Never one to miss an opportunity to tell somebody about my own writing exploits, I chimed right in with the story of *Rescuing Providence*. The other girl in the ambulance said she knew me, her class has a reading club and they might read my book! How do you like them apples!

Stable

I took the last bite from my apple and threw the core out the window. Maybe there will be an apple tree on the spot long after I'm gone. The police had found a woman unconscious in her car near the Temple to Music at Roger Williams Park and called for a medical assist. Engine 11 arrived first, Rescue 1 right behind them.

"Watch out," said Renato, now a member of Engine 11, "she's covered with vomit."

Rob and Seth got the stretcher from the back of the ambulance; Renato did a quick assessment of the girl while I picked up pill bottles and a suicide note from the floor of the car. The stretcher arrived, we got the girl onto it and into the truck and went to work.

"You guys know what to do," I said, trying to make sense out of the mess of belongings I had gathered from her car. I got her name from one of the pill bottles; it matched with the

regi   ther ID. I glanced at the suicide notes, there
wer   st neatly written on an envelope, the others
scra   atever was available: court summonses,
unp   kets, and pieces of scrap paper. I gave the
note

"1   r left hand, EKG rolling," said Renato.
"I   ent, I've got her on 10 liters," said Rob.
I r   spirations were down to 12, her heart rate
180.
"C   an going."
R   and pushed it through the IV.
"N   driver and a guy in back, we have to go."
Se   mbulance, Miles followed in the engine,
and I   nd I stayed in back trying to revive our
patient.

"Bag her."

Rob got the bag-valve device ready, placed the oral airway, and started bagging. A lightning bolt lit the sky as we passed the Temple, thunder close behind. The brilliant light was gone before the thunder roared, plunging the park back into darkness. I picked up the cell phone and watched Rob and Renato work on the girl. Rob assisted ventilations while Renato reassessed vitals and checked the girl's pupils.

"Rhode Island ER," came the voice on the other end of the phone.

"Providence Rescue 1, I've got a twenty-five-year-old female, unconscious, suicide attempt, multiple pills and a note nearby, assisting ventilations, BP 124/68, pulsox 78 percent on room air, glucose 253, two minutes out."

"Thank you, Rescue 1, see you in two."

Seth backed the rescue into the bay, we brought her in. The trauma team took over, me and Renato stayed for a while, assisting ventilations and telling the story again. I was certain she would die. The trauma team wasn't as certain. A few hours later I looked into the room, surprised to see her alive with stable vital signs. She was still unconscious and intubated, but it looks like she will survive. The Providence police deserve credit; she had minutes to live before they found her.

I wonder went through her mind in those last desperate minutes as she sat alone in her car in the deserted park during a thunderstorm, writing goodbye notes and swallowing pills. If she ever reads her words, will they make sense? Will her situation seem as desperate? Will she try again?

Elusive Hummingbird

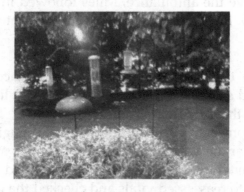

Using the technologically advanced 2003 Verizon "Flip Phone," famed nature photographer Michael Morse captured this magnificent shot of the elusive backyard hummingbird.

"I had to stake out the position," explains Morse, "right next to the refrigerator and food closet."

When asked if all of the waiting was worth it, Morse explains:

"Look at the shot. The exquisite backyard hummingbird is the most elusive of all backyard birds. To the naked eye the green blur next to the red feeder looks like, well, an ordinary blur."

The rest of us can only enjoy the shot and bask in Morse's brilliance.

Close Call

He was lying in his girlfriend's bed and refused to move. When I entered the room he blew his nose on the sheets, then spit onto the pillow.

"What are you doing?" I asked.

He mumbled something and rolled onto his back.

"Why are we here?" I asked.

"He won't leave," said one of the police officers that had responded.

"What's your name?" I asked the man in the bed. Nothing.

"Do you know what day of the week it is?" Nothing.

"Do you know where you are?" Nothing. O for three. So much for my plan to call it a police matter and back out.

"Is he taking any medications?" I asked a woman who I assumed to be his girlfriend. She took a healthy drag from her cigarette, looked in my direction but not at me, and said, "He's supposed to but he's not."

Great.

How to get a three-hundred-pound, spitting, snot throwing, underwear clad, sweaty bear from his lair into my rescue and to the hospital with the least resistance possible?

Force?

Too hard.

Guile?

I'm not that clever.

Trickery?

You bet.

I leaned over the bed, shook the patient firmly, and told him we had to go to the hospital, there is an emergency.

He looked at me with bleary eyes, not comprehending.

"Let's go, we have to go now!" I said, more urgency in my voice. "Something's wrong with you and we can't figure out what!"

We helped him to his feet, put some clothes on him, and walked him through the rain to the rescue.

Too easy.

En route, the patient realized there was no real emergency. He tried to communicate with me but I couldn't understand him. As we sped down I-95 toward Rhode Island Hospital, he became more and more agitated. From the rear windows I noted familiar landmarks. Three minutes away he spit on my stretcher.

"If you spit in here again I'm going to have you arrested."

Two minutes out he started fumbling for the seat belt latch. When he couldn't figure out how to free himself he twisted his one-inch-thick gold necklace in his hands until it tightened around his neck, then he pulled the chain violently up, trying to hang himself.

"You're going to break your chain," I said. The chain miraculously broke in his hands, relieving the pressure to his bulging eyes and letting the blood drain from his beet-red face.

One minute out. He tried to break free of the seat belt by force. I sat three feet away looking for possible weapons. The portable should do the trick if I hit him between the eyes, but what if I missed? The familiar bumps in the road were a welcome relief as we turned onto Dudley Street, one hundred yards from the entrance to Rhode Island Hospital.

Security helped me get him out of the rescue onto one of their stretchers and into the CDU (Clinical Decision Unit), Rhode Island Hospital emergency room's psych ward.

The restraints held. This time.

Speedy Delivery
0700.

"Rescue 1, respond to 465 Baker Street for a maternity, water has broken, eighth pregnancy."

That'll get you moving. Chances of a stretcher delivery increase exponentially after the fifth. Baker Street is approximately three miles from Women and Infants Hospital over some of the bumpiest terrain in Providence. Starting my day with a bundle of joy is not on my list of things to do.

"Speed is of the essence," I said to my driver, Steve. Steve was on hour twenty-four; I was fresh, only fifteen hours in.

"Roger that."

Our patient waited on her porch. When she saw us come over the hill she charged the rescue.

"Not a minute to spare," I told Steve and we were on our way.

"I'm sorry, I soaked your stretcher," said my patient, a lovely thirty-year-old woman.

"Don't worry, the last guy shit in a bucket," I said, flashing back to our previous call.

Through the bumpy streets we sped, delivery imminent. She held on, a real trooper. We delivered her to the hospital, she delivered shortly thereafter.

I love a happy ending.

Doomed
1630 hrs. Called to a tenement house for a man with flu-like symptoms on the third floor. Found said man under a stack of blankets sweating profusely and coughing uncontrollably. Chief complaints:

Coughing blood, no appetite, fever and sweating, irregular heartbeat, sore throat with trouble swallowing, and shortness of breath.

Once inside the incubation chamber otherwise known as Rescue 1, I find my patient just returned from a lengthy stay in Cuba.

I'm doomed.

Symptoms of active TB may include:

Ongoing cough that brings up thick, cloudy, and sometimes bloody mucus (sputum) from the lungs.

Fatigue and weight loss.

Night sweats and fever.

Rapid heartbeat.

Swelling in the neck (when lymph nodes in the neck are infected).

Shortness of breath and chest pain (in rare cases).

Update — 30 Jun 08 0630 hrs.

Tonsillitis. Yay.

In the Air
Responding to a tip-over on I-95, I heard Rescue 6 being dispatched to a house in my district where a woman jumped from the third floor, Rescue 2 to a house a mile away from the house where the woman jumped from the third floor for an injured child, abuse suspected, Rescue 4 sent for a man hit in the head with a crowbar, Rescue 3 had a woman struck by a car, loss of consciousness, Rescue 5 to the bus station for an intoxicated man, and a few out of town rescues sent for the usual assaults, difficulty breathing and seizures.

I swear something strange is in the air sometimes; all hell breaks loose at once. It is the first of the month, but still, this is getting ridiculous!

The guy who rolled his truck self-extricated and escaped any serious injuries. We made him go to the hospital against his will because he was acting like an idiot, head injury suspected.

Fairy Tale

She walked out of the group home, past me, up the steps into the rescue, and sat on the bench, looking out of the rear window. I sat in the captain's chair and waited. Eventually she looked my way.

"I heard you're suicidal."

"That's what they say."

"Who's they?"

"Them in there." She nodded her head toward the house.

"What do you say?"

"What does it matter?"

"What do you mean what does it matter?"

"They say I gotta go for a psych evaluation, I've got to go."

I asked Rob to head toward Hasbro Children's Hospital. Shanaya watched me from her seat, four feet away. She is going to be eighteen in a month.

"What happens when you turn eighteen?" I asked. The state is cutting back and services for children in state custody may be cut drastically. I looked at the young lady seated across from me, tough, determined, and depressed, and wondered how in the world would she survive on her own.

"They mentioned Crossroads."

"You can't go to Crossroads!" I said, sitting up in my seat. Our rescues are called there daily for assaults, overdoses, drunks, and every reason you can think of, and then some. The clientele there is poisoned with chronically homeless people who know the system and how to abuse it. This kid wouldn't have a chance. They would eat her alive.

I sensed she wanted to talk so I pressed.

"Where are your parents?"

"I was adopted when I was four. They gave up years ago. They knew what they were getting into."

"What is that supposed to mean?"

"I'm a lot of trouble."

"How much trouble can you be?" I asked. She was suddenly adorable as her smile lighted her face.

"I stayed out late, cut school, wouldn't listen."

It was probably worse than she let on, but I have a bad habit of placing most of the blame on the parents. Kids are what you make them, for the most part, at least in my world.

"I don't think your parents tried hard enough. Can you go back?"

"They're done with me." She said it with such finality I wondered about the motives of the adoptive parents.

"Is there anybody else?"

"There's seven of us, five boys, two girls." She smiled again. I melted.

"Do you see them?"

We had backed into the rescue bay at Hasbro but I couldn't go in just yet.

Her mood had lightened considerably; she became animated, using her hands as she talked, her eyes sparkling like they always should have.

"We keep in contact on Facebook, all of us, even the baby, she's seven and is going to live with a family in Virginia but she's part of us. We're going to get together as soon as we can."

Rob opened the rear door of the rescue. Shanaya's face dropped, she put the mask back on. I couldn't move for a minute, but she gave me a quick smile, letting me know it was all right, got up and walked into the hospital.

Independence Day
Remember to toast those who have preserved our freedom today. The Greatest Generation, the generations that preceded them, and just as important, our generation.

There is a war going on. If one American soldier dies fighting that war, to that soldier and those close to him, that war becomes just as deadly as any in our history. Remember the families that anxiously await their loved ones' return, remember the families that will wait forever.

I'm proud to be an American, proud of my country, our military, and everybody who works toward making this the greatest civilization in history.

Celebrate our independence on July 4. Travel. Have a cookout. Go to the beach. Enjoy your lives, spend time with friends and family, drink, laugh, and relax. Feel the thunder and beauty of fireworks here at home.

It is an insult to those who have fought and died preserving our freedom to waste it. Enjoy, we've earned it.

9/11 Speech
It is vitally important that we come together on this date to honor those who lost their lives on September 11, 2001. It's hard to believe, but six years have passed, and though the memorials have grown smaller, the painful memories are easier to bear. Some people prefer to block it from their minds, act as if it never happened. That's their choice, not ours. Time marches on; new experiences take the place of memories we once thought would be with us forever. From the depths of sorrow, we find hope. It's a good and necessary thing. Without it, we would be crushed by the weight of sorrow that builds as the years go by.

We've learned to live with the painful memories from that day, but we will "Never Forget!" It is up to us to keep the memory of the fallen alive. This isn't just another day. It's a day when all Americans, and especially firefighters, need to stop and think of what we have, of those who fight for it and of those who died protecting it, and vow to keep their memories alive.

Never forget that every time we put our gear on the truck, we honor the memory of the 343 firefighters who died while doing their jobs six years ago. Every one of us knows we may be asked to risk everything while doing our job. It's not heroic or glamorous or anything else we may have thought it was before we took the oath. It's simply what we do. We are born with it; it's in our blood. Some see it as a curse; most consider it a blessing.

The firefighters who died that day were people like us, proud of their profession, their families, and their ability to save lives and protect property. I'm sure there was a little swagger in their walk that morning when they started their shift, confident they could handle anything thrown at them and somehow walk away. We think the same way; if we didn't, we wouldn't be wearing these uniforms. But with that swagger comes a price. People expect us to save them, and we usually do. Sometimes we don't, and sometimes we die with them.

Thousands of regular citizens showed up for work that day, entered the elevators, sat at their desks, talked at the water cooler, and prepared to start their day. Nothing could have prepared them for what happened next. Most of those who weren't killed instantly waited. For us. We responded. As the world watched the drama unfold on their televisions, helplessly, we responded.

If they thought the job hopeless, they never would have tried it. They thought there was a chance and they marched to their deaths. They didn't go to work that day expecting to die. None of us goes to work expecting to die. Ours is a different profession. We take risks. We work hard and punish our bodies, not because we have a death wish, but because we have a wish that we can make things right when they go horribly wrong, as they did on September 11, 2001. Those who entered the towers thought the poor souls on the upper floors had a chance and they went to go get them.

When the first tower fell, I knew. Before the top floor hit the ground, I said to my wife, "We just lost a lot of firefighters." "Why were they still in there?" she asked.

"They were doing their job."

She looked at me, shook her head, and looked back at the TV, knowing if I were there, I would have been in the tower. It's harder on our families than it is on us.

We owe it to the firefighters who died that day to keep getting on that truck and doing our best, whether it's in New York City, Providence, Warwick, or Cumberland, and to keep doing for them what they did six years ago for the final time. Our duty.

I learned an important lesson that day and the weeks and months that followed. The people we are sworn to protect are worth protecting. We stood together as a nation like nobody could have dreamed possible. We remembered what it meant to be Americans; we stood together, cried together, and together have moved forward. Racial and economic divisions didn't matter, differing political philosophies were irrelevant.

In many ways we've returned to our pre-9/11 mindset, and that is unfortunate, but the togetherness and resolve that existed then still resides in all of us, and comes to the surface when necessary. I know it's there, I remember, and that is what keeps me going.

It's good to be alive, and an honor to be part of the Providence Fire Department, and member of Local 799, but most of all, it's good to be a firefighter.

Downtown, Saturday Night

City Ordinance proposal RB-2112, submitted by Lt. Michael Morse, Rescue 1, 7 July 2008@1123 hrs.

I hereby propose a resolution that will loosen hordes of raging bulls into the streets of Providence at two o'clock in the morning each and every Saturday night or whenever the bars may close.

No Idea

One guy was lying on his back on the sidewalk, gunshot wound to his upper thigh. I took a quick look, was reasonably certain the femoral artery was intact, and walked across the street. Another gunshot victim had run inside the tenement house. He was on his back on the grimy kitchen floor, his leg elevated, blood covering his expensive sneakers and dripping onto the linoleum. I saw two holes in his calf, one in, one out. Rob brought in a backboard, we secured him to it and carried him out of the house toward the rescue. The police had already put up the yellow tape around the front porch, so we had to break through it.

Rescue 5 arrived on scene and took care of the other victim. We took them to Rhode Island Hospital where they told the police that they had no idea who shot them, didn't see anything, no warning, no car, no idea.

Near Miss

0130 hrs.

"Rescue 1 and Engine 14 respond to Bergen Street for an infant injured in a drive-by shooting."

I rolled out of the bunk and was half dressed when Rescue 6 took the call. I waited to hear more.

0133 hrs.

"Engine 14 on scene."

I turned on the light in the office and turned the volume on the radio higher.

0135 hrs.

"Engine 14 to Rescue 6, we have an infant grazed in the head by a bullet, alert and conscious, vitals fine, minimal bleeding."

0140 hrs.

"Rescue 6 transporting to Hasbro."

I turned the light off, lowered the radio, and waited for the next one.

Assholes.

Descent

How could this madwoman drive, I wondered. She rocked in the stretcher, arms folded across her chest, screaming the same phrase over and over, fear filling her eyes. She has a life, I thought, nice home, family, probably a job and friends and everything we all take for granted. The placid, amused expression she had on her face when they took her picture was in stark contrast to the contorted figure on my stretcher. I copied the information and when I went to hand her license back to her, she recoiled and screamed some more.

She has a history of bipolar disorder, depression, and schizophrenia. Something happened this morning; she was at home with her two teenage nieces when she snapped. The girls called 911, we found her at the kitchen table, screaming. She screamed all the way to the hospital and was still screaming when I left.

There is a fine line between psychosis and sanity; I've seen many people cross the line over the years. With proper medication and follow-up care, the mentally ill can be helped and resume some resemblance of normalcy. It is difficult for the families, knowing that at any time their world could be turned upside down.

What causes the descent into madness, and why are only some people afflicted with this curse?

I Wonder

I wonder how it feels to have strangers tell you to calm down, have them reach into your pickup truck and drag you onto a backboard, slap an oxygen mask onto your face, and wheel you into a rescue vehicle.

I wonder how it feels to be held down by those strangers, have large needles stuck into your arms, all the while knowing that you are going to die, but those strangers keep telling you to just breathe and stop fighting.

I wonder how it feels to have your clothes cut off in a room full of doctors, nurses, firefighters, and emergency personnel, and try to answer questions before the sedation medication takes over and a tube is thrust down your throat.

I wonder how it feels to be working at the same hospital that your family member was brought to, and see the chaos that rules during a level 1 trauma, and know that is your cousin fighting for life.

I wonder how it feels to put a gun to the back of a twenty-three-year-old kid's head and pull the trigger, and then shoot him in the face, just to make sure.

I wonder.

Mutual Aid

They were lined up at the kitchen door, waiting for their meds. I walked past them, into an office in the back. The house manager pointed to a man seated in a chair by the back door.

"Take him to the VA."

"Excuse me?"

She handed me the man's information, a piece of paper with his name, date of birth, brief medical history, and medications, and went back to her task.

"He scraped his elbow last night."

The seated man looked at me. The manager looked at me. My partner looked at me. The twenty or so men lined up at the kitchen door waiting for their meds looked at me.

"You can't call 911 for something like this."

"Just give him a ride to the VA," she said, annoyed at my audacity, glaring in my direction, dismissing me.

The patient, a thin elderly man looked miserable, obviously uncomfortable.

"I'll be all right," he said. "I just wanted to clean this up."

The portable radio on my belt continued its nonstop chatter, dispatching rescues to all points of the city. Our six were used up, we had moved on to the surrounding communities, getting mutual aid, leaving those communities with less protection.

"If there is an emergency, there won't be anybody to respond," I said, more to myself because nobody was listening.

"He needs to go to the VA," the manager repeated.

I helped the patient to his feet.

Pool Closed!

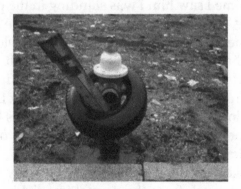

The Potters Avenue Pool will be closed until the next heat wave. Sorry for the inconvenience.

Respect

It's bad enough that they come to Providence, drink themselves to stupidity, tie up our resources because they can't take care of themselves or their friends, and act like complete morons. It gets worse when they vomit on themselves, and the ground next to them and I step in it, and then have to pick their sorry, intoxicated, puke-covered bodies off the pavement. What is intolerable is when their friends, who are unable to look after their own and get them home safely, tell us how to do our job, and when we don't do it to their satisfaction curse and threaten and demand names and on and on and on. Little bastards, I've got kids older than them. They're lucky they aren't mine. But then again, mine would never act that way.

Alive?

I had to look twice at the picture, he didn't belong on the obituary page. He was a young guy, long braided hair, mother dead, raised in foster care, leaving his foster mother, a brother, and two kids without a father.

The last time I saw him I was standing in the pouring rain in somebody's backyard on Prairie Avenue. He had a bullet hole in his head. The rain thinned the trail of blood that ran down his chin and onto his T-shirt, making it look fake. I felt for a pulse, felt the cold skin at my fingertips, no radial pulse, no carotid, nothing. His eyed rolled back in his head. I wanted to close them like they do in the movies but this was a crime scene. I backed out, careful not to trip over the gun that fired the bullet that ended his life.

It's strange, but the picture on the obituary page didn't differ all that much from the mental image I have from the day I determined him dead.

Bedlam

I honestly don't know how they do it. It starts around midnight and doesn't let up until six or so, the living dead roll into the ER, most brought in by rescues, some just waltzing in. The police drag a few over and a couple just appear out of thin air. There is a lot of blood, buckets of vomit, screaming, hysterical laughter, threats of lawsuits, parents calling looking for their kids, and the occasional "real" patient stuck in the middle of all the madness.

I visit four or five times after midnight, adding my share of kooks to the mix. One guy was stabbed in the face, two of my patients were restrained and needed constant observation, one was so intoxicated he couldn't move and another beaten badly, allegedly forced to perform weird sex acts but couldn't remember with whom but did insist on repeatedly showing me her breasts to "see if there were any bruises."

Through it all the nurses, security, doctors, ER techs, and housekeepers keep their cool, treat the patients with dignity, and somehow muddle through, only to do it all again next Saturday night.

Carried Away
If hearing grown men cry makes you sick read no further.

Thirty-eight hours, thirty-four runs. A guy got stabbed in the face. A guy shot himself in the chest. Diabetics, seizures, falls, car accidents, overdoses . . . all part of the deal, I understand.

Toothaches, blisters, and the one that broke the proverbial camel's back at 0545 this morning: the twenty-nine-year-old female who called 911 because she "was tired."

Imagine if you will, me, at 0545 hrs., climbing to the third floor of a tenement house to find a twenty-nine-year-old female, in bed, snuggled under her covers, who simply states, "I'm tired, haven't slept for twenty-two days, and can't walk down the stairs. I need to go to the hospital."

I had Steve bring the stair chair to the third floor. I sat in it and made her carry me down.

Cleaning Up

The housework begins at 0830 hrs. Everybody participates except for some officers, and that's all right, they have done their share of chores. It's one of the things I love about the fire service; scrubbing toilets and mopping floors keeps us grounded.

Every firehouse in the city has the same routine. We don't make it difficult; half an hour usually does the trick. It's not hard, and not a big deal, but it is one of the little things that makes this job so great. If there are other occupations where the menial work is shared up the food chain, I have never heard of them.

Friday night at Rescue 6, stay tuned . . .

The Wall

Sometimes when things aren't going so great in your personal life your job performance tanks. I have some things to deal with on the home front, unpleasant to say the least but ultimately resolvable. The simplest tasks at work now seem insurmountable. Patients are a distraction, reports poorly done, and the only thing I look forward to is quitting time. This is something new to me, and I'm not liking it.

The people keep calling, I keep bringing them to the hospital, and life goes on, but something is missing. I've got a few days off; things should be back to "normal" when I return.

Thanks for standing by.

Thanks

It happens again and again. Just when I think I've had enough, just when one more call might put me over the edge, something happens. It could be an old lady living alone, lonely, sick, and afraid, who doesn't want to bother her family again. It might be a kid who fell off his bike and hurts, but doesn't want to let his friends know how much. Sometimes it's a homeless drunk, destitute, filthy, and nearly hopeless. I never know which one will enter the rescue and make the connection that makes all the trouble worth it.

Often, it's not a connection that keeps me coming back, rather a dramatic save. When a crisis occurs and we respond, well, there simply is nothing better than experiencing what goes on at the scene or in the rescue. The people I work with are the best there is, from the firefighters on scene first, my partner, and the staff at the ER. It's like we enter a different dimension; the people we clown around with, flirt with, torture and goof on suddenly become a team capable of bringing people back from the dead, or preventing further harm and suffering. It never fails to amaze me when everything clicks.

Some people think I'm a great EMT and I let them go right ahead and think it. Truth is, I'm average at best. I'm constantly checking the protocols because I forget things as soon as I read them. If a patient doesn't have pipes, there's a good chance I'll miss the IV. I wouldn't know a dopamine drip from a postnasal drip and have never gotten a rhythm on an asystolic patient. I own most of my success to my coworkers.

Writing has helped me considerably. That people read my words and find a reason to come back, again and again, is truly unbelievable to me. The rescue division in Providence is a thankless position, but we do it voluntarily. We make it hard by working overtime; without that it would be a lot easier to handle. The long hours are what deaden our spirit. Thirty-four hours on, twenty-four off, then thirty-eight on with three days to rest eventually takes a toll. The call volume keeps increasing, but there is no money for more resources and we just keep running. I could give it up at any time and go back to an engine or a ladder company, and believe me, I've been tempted lately.

Time Bomb

She stood in her doorway, hands streaked with blood that poured down from the slashes on her wrists. Before I said a word, she lunged forward, screaming that I was responsible for her brother's death, pointing at my chest with her bloodied finger. The girl's mother stood behind her, tears pouring down her face, mixing with fresh blood from a laceration on her cheek. I stood outside the doorway as a hostile crowd gathered behind me, shouting. I do not understand their language. A Spanish-speaking police officer calmed the crowd while another officer came from inside the house holding a bloody knife. I tried to calm the wounded girl and get her into the rescue to treat her. She was hysterical, violent, and intoxicated. The police had to subdue and transport the girl to the hospital after I stopped her wrists from bleeding. Her mother came in the rescue with me.

En route to the emergency room, she told me the rest of the story. Her son was living with an incurable brain condition. Three days ago he had suffered an attack of some sort, and collapsed where he stood. The family called 911, minutes later an engine company from the Providence Fire Department showed up. The firefighters did what they could, but did not have advanced life-support or transport capabilities. For what seemed an eternity the family waited as the firefighters worked. A rescue from another city showed up twenty minutes later. The family was despondent, the patient deceased.

What happened in the doorway of the family's house was a manifestation of the traumatic experience of three days before. The girl with the bloody hands, overcome by grief, tried to end her life by slitting her wrists. Her mother attempted to stop her. A struggle ensued, the mother was injured, and 911 was called. Luckily, there was a rescue ready to respond.

The city of Providence has five rescue squads on duty at all times. The city has a population of approximately 180,000. During the week that number swells as people come to work. On nights and weekends, the city is full of activity. People come to the city from all over the region because it is a fun, interesting destination where they feel safe. They are not. There are barely enough rescues to meet the demand of the city's residents. Tourists and the workforce stretch the rescue ranks further.

Simply stated, Providence does not provide adequate emergency medical services to the residents and visitors to the city.

It is unfortunate that many Providence residents are poor. A lot of these people have no healthcare insurance. Their primary healthcare providers are the area hospital emergency rooms. When they are sick, they call 911 and are taken by rescue to the emergency room. A large percentage of the rescue runs are for routine medical care that should be provided by a person's doctor. Some people call for a rescue because they have no money for a cab or bus. Others are under the misguided notion that they will get in faster if a rescue takes them. The city's rescues spend a lot of time transporting nonemergency patients.

The homeless present another problem. Day after day the rescues are called for intoxicated persons. Not all homeless people are alcoholics, but enough are to overburden the system. Some call for assistance every day, some twice a day. Frustration mounts when we are transporting one of these patients and hear a call come in over the radio for something serious. We swallow our anger as we hear the dispatcher send an out-of-town rescue to the aid of a child struck by an auto or an elderly person complaining of chest pain. Every day the city's resources are taxed, all the rescues busy, and mutual aid called.

When there is no Providence rescue available, surrounding communities fill the void. Cranston, East Providence, Johnston, and Pawtucket are called daily. Warwick, Central Falls, Cumberland, and others are frequent visitors to the city. These municipalities provide adequate rescue squads for their communities, only to have their protection compromised.

In our business, minutes count. It is impossible to separate the real emergencies from routine calls, and lawsuits are prevalent. The trucks are sent out to whoever calls for whatever reason. Rescues respond to calls from people who have seen ghosts, want pregnancy tests, ran out of their medication, can't open their medication, had a nightmare, a toothache, felt chilly—the list goes on and on. While responding to these emergencies, mutual aid companies are sent for life-threatening problems, such as the suicidal girl's brother. The towns that send Providence their rescues are not getting the protection their taxpayers are paying for.

Throughout it all, the rescue workers maintain the highest level of care and professionalism. When responding to calls that some might call frivolous, we keep in mind that to the person making the call a real emergency exists. Some people are malicious abusers of the system, but most are not. People have been taught that if an emergency occurs, call 911 and help will appear. We are prepared to answer the call, yet frustrated and overwhelmed by the sheer volume of calls.

I started to explain this to the wounded mother in my care, then realized how shallow my words sounded to a person who had lost a loved one, with another in so much pain. I told her I was sorry for her loss, then rode to the hospital in silence.

Alive

I first felt it nearly seventeen years ago. A glow in the distance, cold wind snapping through the tiller cab, not needed to keep me awake, the promise of fire in the distance got my heart pumping. A tillerman on the Providence Fire Department heading toward a two-alarm fire in the middle of a cold winter night is the King of the World. Everything is in focus, the rear of the ladder truck your only responsibility, the wheel in your hands keeping you grounded. Three triple-deckers burning, high-tension wires falling to the ground. The first fire building let go, the front of the building collapsing in front of Engine 12, cutting off their water supply. A fourth home ready to ignite, the vinyl siding already melting to the ground, the family who lived there running out the front door. Me and Danny Brodeur taking a 2½-inch attack line from the rear of Engine 7, Carl Richards squeezing a little more water out of the overburdened pump so we could save the exposure. Lieutenant Healy, standing in the loft of the third fire building before the smoke had cleared, looking toward the east, simply stating, "We'll be here at sunrise."

The same feeling returns, again and again, this time years later, in the loft of an abandoned home on Bowen Street, me and Peter Sperdutti, heavy fire, a window and a charged 1½-inch line. Two other houses burned on either side of us. I was on my third pack, just about spent, as was everybody else on this Memorial Day afternoon. It was us or the fire. The fire lost.

Me and Chris Lisi on the third floor of a filthy tenement on Smith Hill. A woman called because her husband was sick. He took his last breaths as we walked into their apartment. We strapped him onto the stair chair and hauled him out. I called for backup, Engine 7 could be heard in the distance as we put the man on the stretcher and started CPR. I sat in the captain's chair and watched the guys work, IV, O2, EKG, epi, atropine, check pulse, epi, atropine all the way to the ER. They had a pulse when we left. When things quieted down I looked into the back of the rescue, recalling the effort just put forth and felt it again.

A guy with two bullets in his head, still breathing, fighting, dying. We did our thing, got him to the trauma room. He's still alive. I wrote about it and posted the experience on this blog. A few days later, the patient's sister left a comment after reading the post, thanked us for a job well done, and let me know her brother was still alive, still fighting. That same feeling returned, stronger than ever.

I am not a religious man. I don't believe in fate, or destiny. I'm not sure of the existence of God. All that I'm sure of is what I see and feel. The things I've seen in all these years make it difficult to believe in much of anything. What I've felt is a different story. When surrounded by chaos, my life and the lives of others relying on how we respond to the challenge before us, an indescribable calm takes over. It's as if the rest of my time is spent merely existing, it's when crisis hits and the outcome is in question that I truly feel alive.

So Anyway

0800. Responding to a high-rise for a dialysis patient "not feeling well." Engine 15 is first on scene and gives the report.

"Engine 15 to fire alarm, advise rescue we have an unconscious sixty-one-year-old male, assessing vitals."

"Rescue 1, received." I hung the mic back in the cradle.

The address was on the opposite side of the city from Rescue 1, response time about ten minutes. We arrived on scene to find a man barely breathing with a b/p of 80/40. A certified nursing assistant and the patient's best friend stood to the side as we moved the man from his recliner to our stretcher. The CNA offered to clean the patient, who had lost control of his bowels; I didn't want to delay treatment or transport.

"Is there any family?" I asked. Neither answered.

"Does he have any advanced directive paperwork?" Neither knew.

The apartment was barely furnished, just a few pieces of furniture and an old TV. *What did lonely people do before TVs*, I wondered as we moved him out of his home, probably for the last time. Or, are they lonely because of the TV?

The patent's best friend decided he was too busy to come with us to the ER, said he would check later. I told him there may not be a later. He walked away.

I guess people think they will live forever, or if they don't somehow, some way, things will work out for them when their time comes. If only they could be on our side of resuscitation efforts, I think they would get their paperwork done and save themselves a lot of pain and uncomfortable procedures.

Thank You, John

She's ninety years old, a widow, and bleeding uncontrollably from a surgical incision on the right side of her face. She had a "bit of skin cancer" removed earlier in the day.

"Are you my favorites?" she asked, squinting.

"Not yet," I replied.

"I love your haircut," she mentioned to John, my partner tonight. We were both working overtime at Rescue 5. To say that John is follically challenged is an understatement. He bent to help Marcia to our stretcher and she impulsively rubbed his smooth head.

"She is in her glory," said Marcia's granddaughter from a few feet away as the guys from Engine 5, myself, and John helped her along. John was obviously her favorite.

"What is your name?" she asked him.

"John."

She nodded her head, storing the information in her mind with the other ninety years worth of names, faces, and memories.

We controlled the bleeding and headed out. Marcia's granddaughter was unfamiliar with Providence, we transported "code C" so she could follow.

"Is Sarah still with us?" asked Marcia, concerned, looking out the rear windows as the city sped past, backwards.

"We're trying but we can't shake her," I answered, conspiratorially.

"She's good," replied Marcia, laughing.

We arrived at Roger Williams Medical Center a little past midnight. We lifted her from our stretcher to theirs, seldom a gentle experience and this was no exception. Marcia grimaced for a second, then settled in. She took my partner's hand in her own and as we left said, "Thank you, John."

Routine. Uneventful. Extraordinary.

One for Three

The little boy sat on the steps in front of an apartment building, crying. Rich from Engine 10 stood next to him, telling him everything would be okay. A small laceration over his left eye had stopped bleeding, a little scratch on his cheek the only other injury. A neighbor's dog had nipped the boy, probably protective of the puppies she just had.

"Where's your mom and dad?" I asked Pedro. He didn't know. I eventually found the father, pacing back and forth, unable to tell me anything about the boy, he was too upset.

"Your son is fine, he needs you."

The father walked away, said he couldn't handle this.

A police officer came over, shaking his head.

"Can you believe this guy?" he asked.

The boy's grandmother appeared from the crowd, agreed to ride with us to the hospital. I asked her the usual questions, name, date of birth, address; she went one for three.

"You don't know his date of birth?" I asked.

"I have too many grandkids," she said.

"You don't know where he lives?"

"Over there, somewhere," she answered, pointing toward Broad Street.

Pedro sat on the stretcher, his big brown eyes full of tears.

Supply and Demands

Perhaps I was not my usual bubbly self when I showed up at her door at 0430 hrs. Maybe she was annoyed that we used the sirens and lights for a "nonemergency." She could have just been cranky.

"Well, excuse me for calling 911!" she said, full of self-righteous indignation. "I ran out of my inhaler yesterday and need a treatment."

"We'll give you one on the way to the hospital."

"I'm not going to the hospital."

"Why did you call 911?"

"This is unbelievable!"

"Yes, it is."

I put the inhaler together, put some albuterol into the reservoir, and hooked it up to the oxygen. A fine mist came out of one end, the patient, who showed no sign of respiratory distress or any wheezing, breathed it all in. We operate on a replacement policy with area hospitals. What supplies and medications we use we replace at the ER. If we don't transport, we don't replace and must resort to underground tactics to restock our supplies. At four thirty in the morning with twenty hours in and fourteen to go, the path of least resistance looks good.

"Are you done?"

She dropped the empty inhaler on the floor and left without saying a word.

"Rescue 6 in service."

Sneakers

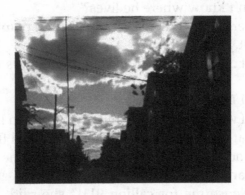

Nothing like the sight of a few pair of sneakers hanging from power lines to warm the old heart! Even an old geezer like me knows that this is a sign that crack dealers are open for business. Maybe a sign saying "Please arrest me" will be here next week.

9/11/08

I don't break out the dress blues too often. Today is one of the days I do. I'll continue to until I am no longer able. Never Forget. I won't.

Today, at a ceremony commemorating the tragic day, union vice president Joseph Mellor and secretary Phil Fiore read aloud the names of the FDNY firefighters and EMS personnel who perished seven years ago. I looked at the people who had gathered, friends, coworkers, and brothers. As the list of names went on, the image of 343 people whose lives were given that day became more clear. If I lost just one of the people next to me this morning the grief would be overwhelming.

God bless the survivors, our thoughts are with you.

I'm proud to belong to Local 799, the Providence firefighters union, and the Providence Fire Department.

Early Start

1106 hrs. Call of the day:

"Rescue 3, respond to 1000 North Main Street for a female who drank too much last night and now feels ill."

Soon after the call I was dispatched to a real emergency, a female who had been drinking all morning and was now intoxicated. Maybe tonight I'll be back for the same female who now feels ill. Maybe this place is making me crazy.

Crushed

The oil truck hit him, threw him off his bicycle, then ran him over. Somehow, he remained conscious. The rear wheels went over his pelvic region, crushing his hips. He could move his toes and I felt a pedal pulse. Shock had set in, his skin was cool and clammy.

"Can you call my girlfriend?" he asked, before asking for something for the pain. I took her name and number and planned to call as soon as things settled down.

Engine 13 had responded along with Rescue 1, six of us, all with a job to do.

"Seth, I need a board and collar." Steve removed the stretcher from the back of the rig while I did a primary assessment. We got him into the rescue, immobilized, vital signs taken, IVs established, high-flow O2 running, 4 mg of morphine in, and got rolling. I picked up the phone. Paul, a firefighter from Narragansett and registered nurse at Rhode Island Hospital, answered on the first ring.

"I've got a twenty-five-year-old male, conscious and alert, stable vitals, struck then run over by an oil truck, diaphoretic, 4 mg morphine on board, we're about two minutes away."

Miraculously, the patient was able to answer all of my questions appropriately. We had him in the trauma room in minutes, all tests underway soon thereafter.

He had just moved here from Boston. He's got a broken pelvis but all vital organs are intact and functioning. I'd like to say that he is lucky, but how lucky is it to be run over by a truck?

Two years ago I responded to the very same location for another man who was run over by an eighteen-wheeler. He too lived to tell the tale.

Ironically, both accidents happened on Terminal Road.

Update—me and Steve checked on our patient a few hours later. He was still in the trauma room, still conscious, broken pelvis but no life-threatening injuries. A few pins and he'll be as good as new, in about a year. His girlfriend and two other friends stood by him. I told his girlfriend that he had asked me to call her but forgot to mention that he did so before worrying about the pain he was in.

"He's a keeper," I told her. He asked our names, and when I told him mine one of his friends asked, "Are you Lieutenant Morse?"

"I am," I said, wondering what I did now.

"I read your book, it was pretty good."

"This will make a good chapter for the next one," I said.

We shook hands and left them to themselves. I couldn't help but think what a great job this is. I am truly blessed.

Over and Out

Whether or not I write about it, *Rescuing Providence* will go on. My part of what happens in the city is small, all things considered. We have six rescues, fourteen engine companies, a special hazards unit, eight ladder trucks, and three chiefs. These thirty-two units are staffed at all times using a four-platoon system. I'm there twenty-five percent of the time, my stories a small sampling of what goes on.

It goes on and on, the calls for help never ending. If you have read this book from the start you have learned a little of what we do. I've kept most of the truly disturbing things out; I never intended to exploit other people's tragedies. Bad things happen, they happen all the time, all over the country, all over the world. This book is my little way of letting people know that there are human beings on the other side of the calls, people with dreams, fears, and problems of their own, people whose lives are affected by what they see and do. We care for you, and we care about you. Even the most jaded of my colleagues is affected by what happens around us. We can't help it, we're only human.

Last week, a needle stuck one of my friends during a routine call. The patient, who is HIV and hepatitis C positive, has no idea that my friend's life has been forever changed. She has started "the Cocktail," a program designed to lower the chances of contracting these diseases. No intimacy, no peace of mind, no peace for six months. They tell us it is imperative we leave the job behind us during our days off. Our minds and bodies need time to heal, process, and rejuvenate so we can do it all again, week after week. There will be no time to heal for my friend; she will be living this nightmare for six months.

Tragically, a seventeen-year-old girl died in a fire last week. The person in charge of Rescue 2 that night was confronted with a nightmare: a helpless person burned over ninety percent of her body. Sometimes we do all we can, try our hardest, but the outcome is preordained. I wonder what went through the lieutenant's mind as she treated the victim, knowing it was already too late. Will she be able to forget, and come back and do it again?

She will. We all will. It's what we do.

Problems

It's three thirty in the morning. I can't sleep, not because I'm not tired, I am. I've responded to twenty-six calls in the last thirty-four hours and have four hours to go. I've got all these stories to tell and nobody to tell them to.

We go through life pretty much oblivious of the drama that surrounds us. We pass thousands of homes, thousands of people, each of them with their own set of problems and joy. A few minutes ago I watched a man dying. He was a hospice patient, or so I surmised from the hospice folder next to his bed. Unfortunately for him, there was no DNR, no Comfort One, nothing even in English. His family gathered around the bed, confused, waiting for something to happen. I couldn't communicate with them. I called the number on the folder and spoke with a hospice nurse. She informed me that the DNR was on file. Great. We took the dying man away from his home, away from his family, and dragged him into the rain and to the hospital where he probably won't see the sunrise.

Problems? Big ones.

A few hours ago I spoke with a woman who has been raped every day for three months by her husband's nephew. The husband allowed it. The woman was forced to submit. Tonight she had enough, tried to end it, and the nephew beat her, then raped her. I have no idea how she summoned the courage to call the police. I can only hope she gets the help she needs.

More problems.

A bunch of stabbings last night, more car accidents than I can count, and the usual drunks and vagrants, all with their own lives, their own circumstances, their own way of coping.

A couple hours to go with this shift, I wonder what will happen next.

The 9th Hole

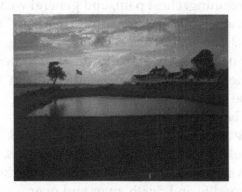

The only thing that could ruin this shot is the fact that it's on a golf course. Somebody defined golf as "a beautiful walk, ruined," which is a perfect description of the debacle that was me at the Warwick Country Club yesterday.

The Plan

She's old, looks it and feels it. Her home does not. Fresh paint, lively flowers, some well-maintained antiques, and a big cat named Mr. Macho filled her space. She told us she was sorry to call and bother us, but she lived alone and was afraid she would die and nobody would know. She didn't want her corpse to foul the space she called home.

Sometimes there is a connection between me and the people who call that is nearly magical. Without saying much to each other a bond was created, and a comfortable friendship formed.

"You look tired," she said.

"I've been here for two days, it's been busy," I replied.

"I'd say a prayer for you but it wouldn't do much good. I don't believe in God."

In combat, somebody said, "there are no atheists in a foxhole." This was no foxhole, but the back of Rescue 1 when you are eighty-seven years old is pretty close. She had some difficulty breathing, chest pain, and general weakness.

"You know what I can't figure out," I asked. "How do you explain cats? The little beasties actually love us, and I'm not talking about the genetic need to suck up to people so they will feed them. They really have affection in their hearts. That can't be an accident."

"Do you believe in evolution?" she asked.

"I believe there is a plan, and I don't think any of us is capable of fully understanding what that plan is. I know how I feel when I see the leaves turning, how the cycle of life plays over and over, life and death, over and over."

"I'd like to believe there is something else," she said.

"There is."

We transferred her from our stretcher to the hospital bed, the nurse took my report, and my job was done. I looked at my patient as I was leaving. She waved me over to her side.

"It may be inappropriate, but I think I love you," she said with a mischievous grin.

There is a plan. There has to be.

Breathe

He didn't look right. His mother cradled his limp form in her arms and tried to explain what happened.

"We heard a crash from the bedroom, he was under the dresser!"

I looked into the bedroom in question. A full-sized dresser stood against a wall, somebody had righted it after it fell, its drawers on the floor in front of it and a big TV perched on top. The baby rolled his eyes back, unresponsive.

"Did he cry when it happened?"

"No, he was quiet."

We were on the third floor.

"Get the papoose ready, we're coming down," I said out loud. Engine 14 was there to assist, I was sure somebody would be at the rescue getting things done. The eighteen-month-old baby's mom didn't want to let go, I let her carry the boy to the rescue. There she had to step aside. Although we had a lot of work to do I thought it best she stay in back with us. She knelt next to the stretcher while we worked. We worked around her. It wasn't that hard. The baby cried a little while we restrained him. I was relieved to hear something. There is no worse sight than a still, restrained, bluish grey infant in the back of a rescue.

"Let's roll."

Jermaine hit the gas and we were on our way to the trauma room at Hasbro.

"Do something! Hurry up!" said the boy's mom from the bench seat, frantic.

"We all have kids of our own, we're doing everything we can," said Ariel, my partner for the overtime shift. He said it gently, looking the mother in the eye. It worked, she relaxed.

The baby needed an IV. Ariel is not assigned to rescue, his usual spot a firefighter on Engine 11. I've worked with him a few times; he's calm, competent, and more than willing to do the job. Asking somebody to start an IV on an unresponsive infant in a moving truck in front of a panicked mother is not something I do lightly. Alas, we all have a job to do, and I was not doing mine.

"I need an IV."

"I'll get it."

Simple. I moved from the infant's side, sat on the captain's chair, and called the ER at Hasbro.

"Providence Rescue 6, we have an eighteen-month-old male, semiconscious, responds to painful stimuli, no obvious deformities with a heart rate of 140 and 128/96, respirations 40 and shallow, pulsox 98 percent with blow-by O2."

Ariel and Hans, another firefighter from Engine 14 who had joined us, were wrapping up the IV and were checking the baby's glucose level.

"IV established, he's restrained, BG of 184, ETA four minutes."

"See you in four."

The baby stopped breathing.

"Is he all right?" asked the mom.

For what seemed an eternity the little guy lay on the stretcher, motionless. Ariel shook him, I squeezed his little hands . . . nothing. As I reached for the pedi bag valve mask and got ready to start CPR, the most beautiful sound filled the back of the rescue, a baby's crying. Not loud, not in earnest, but crying nonetheless.

"He's fine," I told the mom. "He is injured, but things are under control. We'll be at the hospital in a minute."

A minute later we backed into the bay at Hasbro. The trauma team was ready, I gave my report, and they took over.

Then I started to breathe.

Still Walking

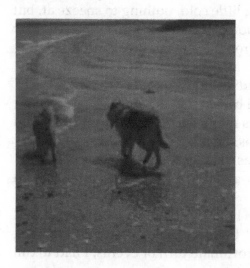

And they really never stopped . . . they just kept on walking.
  Man, I miss those dogs.

Assisted Living

They call it assisted living. I don't know what to call it. A fifty-one-year-old male sits in his apartment, drinking vodka, smoking Pall Malls, and taking Vicodin. He has COPD, diabetes, and a host of other problems. Because he is "disabled" he's allowed to live in the high-rise with the elderly. He abuses his pain meds so a med tech, whatever that is, is hired by the facility to administer medication to him.

Tonight, our hero was difficult to waken; the "med tech" decided he had to go to the hospital. Enter the anti-heroes from Rescue 1.

Perhaps a little history will help clarify the tale I'm about to tell. I've been here since 0700. It's now 2135 hrs. I'll be here a while longer, and that is fine, it's what I do. I've taken ten or so people to the hospital today, none sicker than myself. I'm battling an annoying little cold, nothing to sneeze at, but really no reason to stay home from work either, or call 911 for a ride to the emergency room for what, I really don't know.

We enter the man's apartment to find him smoking, conscious and alert, and a little buzzed. The "med tech" informs me the man will be taken to the emergency room for an evaluation and hands me his list of medications. I asked him what day today was, he answered. I asked if he knew where he was. He did. I asked if he knew who was president. He knew. I asked if he wanted to go to the hospital. He did not.

I cannot enter a man's home and force him to leave, I said to the "med tech." Well then, she said, not quite knowing what to make of this unfortunate turn of events, I had to call somebody!

It seems that the somebody she called to wipe the ass of her resident was tired of wiping asses. The "med tech" was unable to wash her hands of her problem, and Rescue 1 returned to service.

Sharing

He shares the bathroom with six others. When it was his turn something happened; maybe he turned the wrong way and slipped, maybe his "bad knee" finally gave out, maybe his heart finally gave up. He could have overdosed or had a stroke, we really had no way of knowing until we found a way in.

He was crumbled up against the in-swinging door. Not a big man, but big enough to make things difficult. If we forced the door, we would hit his head when the door swung in. If we broke the lock and gently pushed we could do further damage to his c-spine.

As minutes passed and the peanut gallery grew more impatient, we forced the door with a Halligan tool and Miles, the skinniest among us, slipped in. He had to step into the shower, then behind the patient. He moved him enough so I could fit in. I normally avoid touching walls in these places but there was no way around it. I squeezed through the tight opening and into the shower, then worked around the patient and straddled the toilet while positioning the patient.

He was semiconscious and semi-naked. Possible vagal reaction? We checked for trauma, there were no obvious signs, no drug paraphernalia, BG 115, 120/60, HR 76. We carried him to the rescue, worked him up, and brought him in. He was talking normally before I left the hospital.

I spent a lot of time in the communal bathroom getting him out. I spent just as much time at the communal bathroom at the fire station washing the itch off.

Impossible

"What does it take to be an EMT?" he asked, innocently enough. It was his first time in the back of an ambulance, strapped to a longboard with a c-collar in place, immobilized. He looked around as best he could, his mind active, considering the possibilities.

"You have to go to school, learn about how the body works, how it breaks, and how to put it back together. That's the basic level. Then you have to go to more school, learn how the heart works, how to fix it when it isn't working right, and a ton of other stuff. That is the cardiac level. Then you can go back to school, learn even more, and become a paramedic."

"Is it hard?"

I looked at him, lying there on the backboard after he crashed his car through a fence. His right leg lost all feeling, a result of his progressive form of multiple sclerosis. He couldn't feel the gas or brake pedal, couldn't move his leg even if he could. It took a lot of courage to steer through the fence instead of continuing on.

At eighteen, I'm sure he considers his disease a temporary setback; how could he think otherwise? It takes years of disappointment and frustration before you give up hope. Decades.

"It's hard," I said.

It's impossible, I thought.

I love being wrong.

In Case You Missed It

Morse makes a brilliant move, moves from the couch to the bed, takes an Ambien from his pouch, and starts to chew. Pedroia, the bald-headed, potbellied MVP candidate, whacks a two-out single, Morse spits out some Ambien juice and turns up the volume. Big Papi walks to the plate, swinging the same bat he carried to first the last time he was up, and weakly grounded out. Shouting tough love from his suburban bedroom, Morse encourages the slumping Ortiz . . .

"You're going to look awfully funny with that bat sticking out of your ass, Little Papi!" screams the bed coach as Papi digs in. Spurred on by the noise from the bedroom, Ortiz launches one over the wall, the crowd goes wild, Morse rips the covers from his bed, waves Auntie Rose's homemade quilt above his head like a championship banner, and runs naked through the house screaming "PAPI, PAPI, PAPI!"

Bottom of the ninth; Morse returns to his bed, unwilling to jinx the comeback. JD "Stop it, my back hurts!" Drew steps in. Morse shouts more words of wisdom . . .

"Quit crying, Nancy, and get a hit, for Christ's sake!" Drew listens and launches a single, the winning run scores, and Morse finally relaxes, knowing that without him, the season would be over.

The lights go out until Saturday, giving Morse plenty of time to prepare.

Loss

He's old now, closer than ever to infinite eternity. His mind is gone, the brilliant thoughts that once sprang to life as written words confused and meaningless, just syllables uttered to a stranger who came into his life too late to appreciate him, and possibly learn from him. I sat across from him in the back of Rescue 1, mesmerized, his eyes still burning with intensity as he uttered strange words, some in Spanish, some English. The words had a cadence when he spoke them, a rhythm and maybe some kind of message. His eyes bored into mine as he said over and over, "Stink, stank, stunk." He would change into a foreign language and utter more words in the same way, earnest, almost desperate.

At first I was amused, things like this don't happen every day. As the ride progressed, sadness crept in. Sadness for the man, and what was lost, sadness for myself as I envisioned a similar fate, and sadness for those close to him, who had experienced his intellect before Alzheimer's disease invaded his mind.

This is a strange existence.

Edwin Honig, poet and translator, has published ten books of poetry, eight books of translation, five books of criticism and fiction, three books of plays. He has taught at Harvard and Brown, where he started the Graduate Writing Program, and has received numerous awards from the Guggenheim Foundation, Mishkenot Sha'ananim, the National Endowment for the Arts, and the Academy and Institute of Arts and Letters. In 1986 he was knighted by the president of Portugal for his work in literary translation, and in 1996 by the king of Spain. He is emeritus professor at Brown University.

Edwin is a great, powerful man who will leave this earth soon. He leaves us not only with the gifts of his own writings and translations, but also the planted seeds of thought and inspiration in the minds of countless students and others who enjoy his work.

Alzheimer's disease and other manifestations of dementia are cruel, devious companions for those unfortunate enough to be saddled with the affliction. It is far worse for those left caring for the victims.

I do not know Edwin, other than a brief moment where I was responsible for his well-being. I hope that in some way he knows and finds comfort knowing I found his work, and that he leaves an indelible impression on me that will last a lifetime.

I think that on some level Edwin understands and approves of my writing about him here. Writers have a need to be read and understood. I understand, Edwin. I understand.

An inclusive volume of Edwin Honig's poetry, titled *Time and Again: Poems 1940–1997*, is available at xlibris.com/timeandagain.html.

Healthcare?

It is my pleasure telling you about life here in the homes and streets of Providence. I hope I've painted a vivid picture for those of you who don't get to experience firsthand what it is that we do. It is a noble calling, something I am honored to be part of. When my time on earth comes to a close, the part of my life I'll be proudest of will no doubt be my time spent as a Providence firefighter.

When I swore the oath of office, I had only a vague idea of what the next twenty-plus years of my life would entail. I did know that I would be put into precarious situations, witness heartbreaking incidents, and be challenged to perform at a level that I hoped resided within me. Looking back, I can honestly say I've met the challenge, and continue to do so, and will continue to do so for as long as the city of Providence pays me.

Honor. It isn't a word I use lightly. In the end, it is all we have.

Society is full of uncertainty; the economy is in trouble, fuel unstable, healthcare in question. Right now, the administration of Providence has informed ten thousand people whom the people of Providence employ that their healthcare provider will be changed from Blue Cross to United effective January 1, 2009. My union, Local 799, brought representatives from United to meet with us and explain the changes that are forthcoming. We are ready, willing, and able to do our part and facilitate the transition that was thrust upon us. We found that there is no plan, no answers, no idea of what to expect until it happens, and then we can crawl through the morass of red tape and bureaucracy, not knowing if our family doctors will participate, our medications are covered, or, well, anything until it happens.

Just my opinion, but a pretty lousy way to implement needed change in our healthcare system.

The people of Providence benefit from the honorable service of their police and fire departments every day. It is an honest trade, our integrity, blood, sweat, and sacrifice for their tax dollars. A contract, honorable, solid, and just. It is the backbone of our society.

When we lose that backbone, as the administration of Providence is currently doing, the foundation cracks. Although the people that were elected by the residents of Providence are doing their best to undermine the integrity of our beliefs, we, the people doing the work, will remain strong.

Sometimes It's Easier

"I could hit Rhode Island Hospital with a rock."

"I don't go there."

"Why did you call us?"

"I need to go to the hospital."

"I'll take you."

"Not that one."

And so it goes. My patient, an eighty-five-year-old great-grandmother, insisted on being taken across the city to Miriam Hospital, a smaller place on the east side. Rhode Island and Miriam are affiliated, the same doctors, record keeping, security.

"You'll have to find another way."

"They took me last night."

She had been released from Miriam Hospital a few hours ago. At 0100 hrs., a Providence rescue unit took her from her home, bordering the parking lot of Rhode Island Hospital's emergency room, to Miriam. I have no idea why. Sometimes it's just easier.

Mondays are nonstop, the calls just keep coming. My portable radio continued to transmit, a Cranston rescue to Broad Street, a Smithfield rescue to Admiral Street, East Providence to Kennedy Plaza. All the while, her family members started to pour into the little house.

"Why ain't they takin' her?"

"I don't know."

"They took her last night."

"Those guys weren't assholes."

I suggested they call for a private ambulance. They did. We waited. The family continued to grow. We continued to wait. The patient was in no distress, normal vital signs, possibly dehydrated, according to the paperwork from Miriam, a few hours old.

"I must be an asshole," I muttered forty-five minutes later as we loaded her into the truck and took her to Miriam.

Ten Runs, One Emergency

"We have to get back to the station, I've got to go."

"You're not going to shit your pants like the last guy, are you?"

"Maybe."

It's a three-mile trip from the Rhode Island Hospital emergency room to the Allens Avenue Fire Station. ETA six minutes. I could probably make it. Everything was going great, light traffic, perfect weather conditions, no road construction in sight. I could see the Promised Land in the distance, a little more than a minute away. I started to relax.

"A train!"

"You have got to be kidding."

"It's the coal train, slowest moving locomotive on the Eastern Seaboard!"

"Oh, my, God."

The railway gates closed, blocking our approach. Lights flashed, the train approached Allens Avenue at 2 mph. Doomed.

"Turn around, we'll backtrack to the one way, circle around the X-rated bookstore, go up the one way down and over the railroad tracks."

"Let's roll."

As we approached the one way and were about to put on the warning lights and sirens, a battalion chief approached.

"BOGEY AT 12 O'CLOCK!"

"You have got to be kidding!"

I curled my toes, waved to the chief as we passed his vehicle, now headed away from the Promised Land.

"Stop at the Burger King!"

"I'm on it!"

Mark wheeled Rescue 1 around and headed toward the burger joint. Thirty seconds away the pain in my abdomen subsided.

"I think I can make it, keep going."

"Are you sure?"

"I can do this. I can."

The station was around the next bend, salvation moments away. I saw it in the distance, a beacon, a ray of light, the most beautiful thing I had ever seen. We roared onto the ramp, I rolled under the opening overhead door and duckwalked to the restroom, just in the nick of time.

What a day. Ten runs, one emergency.

Inspiration

I'm running out of gas about now, the minions of Providence have kept me running. Called to a house on Elmwood Avenue, a boardinghouse, not known for the upscale clientele. Trudge up the stairs to one of the rooms, heavily fortified and completely unsanitary, to find a fifty-nine-year-old male hunched over in an easy chair racked with pain.

"What's the matter?"

"I slept in my chair, now my back hurts."

"Get up and stretch."

"Can't. Broke my ribs."

"Well, sit and stretch."

"Can't, broken vertebrae."

I took a closer look. The visor on his "Dewey, Sueem & Howe" cap laid low on his forehead. A handsome black guy looked up at me through eyes filled with pain.

"Come on, we'll get you to the hospital."

"My doctor is at Miriam."

Here we go again. I started to tell him there was no way I was going to take him across town to Miriam when I saw his medications. HIV+.

"How long have you had HIV?"

"Since '83."

Miriam Hospital has a program where they do great work with AIDS and HIV+ patients. A crosstown trip wouldn't kill me. We loaded him up the best we could, broken ribs and vertebrae are tough injuries to work around. He was a trooper, only complained a little.

Inspiration comes from the strangest places. This time, in the back of Rescue 1, two guys from different worlds talking about the Celtic and Laker years of the eighties. He was a Lakers fan, me, the Celtics. Didn't matter, it was as if Magic and Bird were in the rescue with us.

"I remember when I heard about Magic," I said. "Thought he was a goner."

"Thought I was a goner." He smiled and reminisced. Magic Johnson. Larry Bird. Lew Alcindor. Robert "the Chief" Parish. Worthy, Johnson, and all the rest. I felt like I was with an old friend watching the game and having a beer.

Turns out he's a Vietnam-era combat wounded veteran. Marine Corps. Didn't talk much about that, one of the security guards at Miriam served with him and told me. Marines. Semper Fi. They mean it.

I wonder if the other folks at Miriam saw a destitute former addict with HIV and not much else. I hope not.

Don't Mention It

It used to be when somebody got shot we would talk about it. Who responded, where were they shot, how many times, were they breathing, how much blood, were you in danger?

The news was sure to follow the story for a few days, the camera crews would fight for position on the sidewalk as we tended to the wounded. Follow-up stories would air for days, the patient's condition, the police investigation, the family's response.

Now, somebody has to die to get a mention, even then it is fleeting, just a word or two tucked away on the back page, a sentence read on the second segment of the local news, not mentioned again at eleven.

We don't bring up the details anymore, and nobody back at the station asks about it. We just clean the truck and get ready for the next call.

A six-year-old was shot in the abdomen during my days off this week. I heard the story on the radio, the night before the election, third or fourth story into the newscast. I quickly forgot about it until yesterday.

I was working with Mark, who was working overtime on my shift. We drove past the location where the kid was shot. Mark told me, "We had that kid." I instinctively knew what he was referring to.

"What happened?"

"Little kid got shot in the stomach and his uncle shot in the arm. The kid is still in critical condition."

Mark doesn't say much so I had to drag it out of him. He reluctantly continued.

"The kid didn't even cry. We put him on oxygen and after a minute he raised his hand. He was the most polite kid I've ever seen. He said, 'I'm breathing okay, I don't need this.' His mother was in the rescue, talking to her boyfriend in Puerto Rico. 'Take care of your kid,' I said, 'He needs you.' She kept on talking. I held his little hand on the way to the hospital while she sat on the bench. We were getting closer to the hospital when his eyes started fluttering. I told Mike we were losing him."

"He might not make it," I said.

"I know," said Mark, turning away from me. He didn't mention it again.

New Friends

At five o'clock Saturday morning two women and three Providence police officers stood next to the rescue and squad cars in front of a triple-decker off Broad Street. The women, both around thirty-five, were dressed to kill: high heels, tight, short dresses, beautiful hair, just right for a night on the town. One of the women was covered with blood that ran from the top of her head. She had been hit over the head with a bottle. The other woman knew the person who committed the crime and was trying to relay that information to the police officers.

"I know who did it," she explained. "Why won't you listen to me!"

"Why don't you worry about your friend who's bleeding to death instead," said one of the officers.

"Come on, we have to take her to the hospital," I said, helping the bleeding woman into the rescue.

"What happened to you?" I asked her. She was all smiles between the rivers of blood that ran down her face.

"I don't speak English," she answered, still smiling.

"Get in the truck, I need a translator," I said to the other one.

"I want to go home," she replied. "My car is over there. I just want to go home."

"That's just great. Your friend is bleeding to death over here and you want to go home. What the hell kind of friend are you anyway!"

I shook my head in disgust and started to close the door. The other woman stopped me.

"I'll go."

"Nice. Unbelievable."

Jen tended to the victim's wound and I started the report, one woman translating for the other. They sat next to each other on the bench seat. Slowly, the story unfolded.

They had been at a nightclub on Broad Street. When the club closed they went to a party at one of the houses nearby. Fun was had by all until somebody decided she wanted to fight. The woman who sat bleeding in my truck ended up being the victim.

"I didn't want to get involved but she needed somebody to help her," said the translator.

"That's the least you could do, that's what friends are for," I said, in my best *Father Knows Best* voice.

"I guess, but I don't even know her. She was with some other people who left early."

Talk about feeling like an ass. Add kidnapping to my resume.

An hour later I returned to the ER with another patient. The two women were still waiting, sitting next to each other, talking. I offered to give the translator a ride back to her car. She declined, said her new friend needed her.

That's what friends are for.

Quiet Thursday

Triple stabbing? It's Thursday afternoon, for Pete's sake! Just when the minions of Providence lull me into a false sense of security with calls for "chest pains" that are actually the common cold, "severe lacerations" that have to be squeezed to get a drop of blood, "CVAs" that are two-day-old headaches, "unresponsive males" that are the daily drunks, and "severe abdominal pains" that are actually cramps, some maniac stabs three eighteen-year-olds in front of a middle school.

My patient had a two-inch stab wound to his lower left abdomen, diaphoretic and going downhill but didn't want to go to the hospital, another rescue got a kid with truly severe lacerations to his arms, and a third victim is still unaccounted for.

After explaining the severity of his injuries to my patient, something like "quit being an idiot, you've been stabbed," we carried him to the rescue and transported him to Rhode Island Hospital. He was in the trauma room last time I checked.

Mouse Trap
"You were bit by a mouse?"
    "Right on my foot."
    "Did you see the mouse?"
    "No, but I know it was a mouse."
    "How do you know?"
    "Because my cat chased him into the box."
    "Did the cat follow him in there?"
    "No, he didn't fit."
    "Why did you put your foot into the box if you knew there was a mouse in there?"
    "I didn't think mice bit."
    "Maybe it was a rat."
    "No, it was a mouse."
    "Are you sure?"
    "Positive."
    "Baby rat?"
    "Mouse."
    "Get in the truck."

Enough
There is talk of closing fire companies in Philly and elsewhere and adding ambulances. Budget cuts. Let's enable those unwilling to care for themselves, the looters, pickpockets, and leeches of society, let's keep sending ambulances to every fool who calls 911 for a toothache, a sore throat, a mouse bite, and a free ride. Let's continue wiping the asses of those people with no conscience, no scruples, and no backbone.

We might as well throw in the towel now, folks, Karl Marx was right.

Response times apparently don't matter to those whose primary purpose is keeping the "people" happy. No matter that the mob is suffocating independence, free will, responsibility, and work ethic. Keep the drooling masses happy, just continue providing services and never tell them no.

Tell that to the people hanging from their windows waiting for a ladder company to save their lives.

Or their families when they claim the bodies.

Business as Usual

She sat in the Amtrak police office at Providence Station, blood dripping from her lip onto the front of her jacket. Two Amtrak police officers and a Providence cop asked questions while I waited to transport her to the emergency room.

Her estranged husband had broken into the apartment that she shared with their daughter, punched her in the face, then kicked her in the back of the head once she had fallen. He left then, after making his point. What that point is I'll never know. The couple's eight-year-old witnessed the assault and isn't talking. How the two ended up at the train station I have yet to figure out.

She sat next to her mom in the back of Rescue 1 as we rode to the hospital. She smiled at me between bites of an enormous chocolate chip cookie that a police officer bought for her. I noticed that she stashed half of the cookie in her jacket pocket, maybe for later, maybe for a friend, maybe for her mother when things quieted down.

She didn't seem upset by all of the commotion. I think that made it worse.

Our World

With barely a year on the job I participated in an Incident Stress Debriefing following the death of two toddlers who burned to death at three in the afternoon one bright, sunny Sunday. Twelve firefighters sat in a room and talked about the incident, one at a time, venting, I guess. When it was my turn, I simply stated that I did all I could, fate had other plans. Nobody pressed, the discussion went on.

One guy, a twenty-year veteran highly respected firefighter, started to tell his story. He didn't make it through the first sentence, broke down in tears instead. The old-timers waited for him to compose himself, I fidgeted in my seat, uncomfortable and a little confused. I didn't understand how a person with so much experience could be so devastated by something that had only a minimal effect on me. That firefighter never made it back to the trucks; he retired soon after. I haven't seen him since. Some people leave the job and never look back; others hang around for a while before quietly disappearing from station life.

It has taken decades, but I finally understand. My mind stores everything, whether or not I choose to acknowledge what lies lurking in the shadows. Horrific memories become a part of my subconscious mind, left to fester and decay but never go away. The only way to free myself is to let those images out of their prison, talk about it, let them go. Problem is, I have a hard time talking about these things.

As you may have noticed, I have no problem writing about them.

Whole Again

"Nothin' but a dead body up there." The man on the porch referred to his brother, an active alcoholic who has been fighting a losing battle with his disease for years.

It's over, I thought. No more late-night calls for an unconscious male, no more arguing with him, convincing him to go to the hospital and get some help, no more carries. Though saddened by his demise, the remaining family must have felt some relief. This day was long overdue. There is a distinct difference between living and existing, and he had crossed the line a long time ago. His existence came to an end the day after Thanksgiving.

I entered the home, probably for the last time. Some familiar faces milled about, making room for me as I slowly walked up the stairs. A woman stood outside the room at the top of the landing, tears running down her face.

"I'm sorry," I said and walked past her into the bedroom. He was lying on his back, eyes open, dead. Forty-five years on this earth done, not all of those years as poorly lived as the most recent. His mother sat next to him, holding onto what was left. She remembered the baby, the boy, the young man. Once there was hope and a promising future, now just a dead body and remorse.

The body finally joined the spirit in death.

Another Year
With a little luck I'll have made it through another year. There are still ten-plus hours to go in 2008. With an Alberta Clipper roaring through the heart of Providence as I write this, and New Year's Eve upon us, the chance that those hours will pass uneventfully are slim. I just hope that nobody gets hurt.

December has been a tough month for the people of Providence. A couple of kids were murdered at the downtown clubs, an eleven-year-old girl fell through a glass-top table and bled to death, a six-year-old died at home for unknown reasons, a dozen stabbings, lots of shots fired, and numerous occupied house fires made life difficult for a lot of families.

Members of the Providence Fire Department respond to these and thousands more incidents every year. Lives are saved, property protected, and the citizenry of the city kept as safe as possible. I speak for every member of this department when I say I wish we could save them all. God knows, we try. Sometimes everything we have just isn't enough.

In spite of all this, and the political dissent, outdated equipment, and insufficient resources, one thing keeps me coming back.

Happy New Year, Brothers and Sisters, and stay safe.

Stragglers

Despite some nasty weather the party went on. New Year's Eve was memorable for a lot of people, and better off forgotten by others. Six revelers crossed my path last night, lonely stragglers abandoned by their friends, left to battle the elements and fend for themselves. The first we found barefoot in a snowbank, semiconscious and semi-dressed. How she ended up alone, heavily intoxicated and lost, is a mystery. We wrapped her in some blankets and took her to the ER. A little later a lost soul wandered into the lobby of a downtown apartment building. Another one without a coat on a frigid (8 degrees, 40 mph wind gusts) New Year's Eve. He was almost as drunk as the guy on the other end of the phone he handed to me. Both were lost. We took him to the ER.

There was the stunning twenty-four-year-old at the Westin. Her dress and shoes probably cost more than my car. No idea what happened to her — we found her curled up in a ball, lying in a puddle of her own vomit on the floor in the lobby. The obligatory combative twenty-year-old male was next. He was in the back of a police cruiser, unconscious, until he got on the stretcher and turned into the Incredible Drunken Hulk. The Incredibly Disgruntled Rescue Guy quickly put to rest any idea of insurrection that may have crossed the drunken boy's mind; he didn't make a peep after the initial, short-lived outburst.

A restaurant employee mysteriously appeared at the Providence Place Mall at 0500, drunk and disoriented. He was actually pretty funny. Had to take him to the ER anyway. That makes five. I know there was six. I can't for the life of me remember the sixth one. I'll probably have a flashback when I least expect it.

Speaking of the ER, the people there were amazing as always, keeping things positive in the midst of the circus. The night shift set up a buffet in the break room and invited some of us to partake in some of the goodies. It was a welcome respite, away from the sea of stupidity that threatened to drown us.

And speaking of stupidity, where were the friends of the "stragglers" who continued to pop up as the New Year progressed? These kids are supposedly more connected to each other than ever before. I never lost a friend at a party, not once, and I didn't have GPS, cell phones, text messaging, MySpace, Facebook, YouTube, or a Wii. We just had each other, and that was enough.

I Know

"Besides the allergic reaction do you have any other medical problems?"

The question is part of our patient assessment, one we ask every patient under our care. Beatrice, a forty-four-year-old woman suffering from a possible allergic reaction to hair detangler, lay on my stretcher, oxygen mask covering her swollen but pretty face and answered quietly.

"I have an underactive thyroid, acid reflux, and . . . multiple myeloma."

I stopped writing and took a closer look. Of course, I thought. Her close-cropped hair was in stark contrast to the images displayed in the family portraits that decorated her living room. The swelling in her face wasn't a result of the allergic reaction, rather a prolonged battle with cancer. I've seen the look before, close to home.

"You mentioned the multiple myeloma last," I said to her.

"I know."

Ninety-nine out of a hundred people would have told me about the cancer before I had two feet in their door. It is all-consuming, a diagnosis as frightening as that, tough to get out of your mind.

"You are going to survive," I said, not really sure why I said it.

"I know."

Communication

Three of his twelve kids hovered around him, making sure we did everything right.

"He's a great dad," one of his daughters said as we gently secured him to the stair chair.

"Obviously," I replied, noting the concern on the family's faces. It's gratifying to see a family come together at times like these, a true testament to the character of the patient entrusted to my care.

He had a brief period of unresponsiveness before we arrived. His blood pressure was high, 168/120, his heart racing at nearly 150 beats a minute. Skin warm and dry, he must be fighting an infection of some sort.

"How are you feeling, Joe?" I asked.

"He has Alzheimer's," said another of his daughters. "He comes and goes now. Right now he's not aware of anything."

The family members stood back as we wheeled out of his home, the place he raised twelve children. I imagined the living room as it used to be, orderly chaos, kids' things, books, crayons, and toys rather than medical equipment and empty space.

He met his wife in Portugal some sixty years ago. He was a fisherman, she said he was special. More kids arrived as we got ready to transport him to the hospital. He managed to look me in the eye as I carried him down the freshly shoveled front stairs and into the cold.

"How long has he had Alzheimer's?" I asked the daughter who accompanied us in the rescue.

"About a year and a half," she replied, leaning over to hold his hand. He stared intently at his daughter as we drove.

"Have you been able to communicate with him at all?"

"We communicate just fine," she said. "We're not ready to let him go, not yet."

"Joe," I said, shaking his shoulder from my seat behind him. "Are you in any pain?"

I didn't think he would answer but you never know.

"He can't hear you," said his daughter, never breaking eye contact with her dad.

"He was born deaf and mute."

Great dad indeed.

Strength and Experience

He sat in a chair in the corner of a once-white bathroom, surrounded by attendants, skin as white as the walls were before being covered with his blood. The coppery taste in my mouth and sticky feeling on my skin connected me with this patient, whether I wanted it or not. His neck was sliced open, blood oozing from the one-inch laceration that missed his jugular by a fraction of an inch. His right arm was split open, just missing a major artery. His left arm bore the brunt of the self-inflicted attack, blood pumped from the wound in perfect rhythm with his rapid heartbeat. He must be right-handed, I thought, applying pressure to stop the blood loss.

Somebody from the staff at the psych ward inflated a blood pressure cuff above the wound, probably saving the kid's life. A flow of water continued to run from a sink in the corner, overflowing, mixing with the pool of spilled blood that covered the floor. Sheets were thrown down, absorbing some of the mess, turning the starched and bleached bed coverings into pink sponges. They squished as I walked over them, toward the patient. He was fading fast, hypotensive, major blood loss and losing consciousness.

We dragged the chair he sat on while carving himself toward the door, lifted him onto our stretcher, and wheeled him past the secured doors toward Rescue 1, three floors below. From there it was business as usual, the chaos we left behind would sort itself out eventually, I was in my zone, with people I knew I could count on.

We replaced the 22-gauge IV somebody from the hospital had started in the kid's bicep with a large-bore IV, loaded him up with ringers and O2, and rolled toward the trauma room at Rhode Island Hospital. The fluids and O2 did him good, he became combative en route, but not nearly strong enough to do any real harm. The crew from Engine 10 helped restrain him during the five-minute transport.

We transferred care to the level 1-A trauma team that had assembled, BP 83/30, HR 140 or thereabouts. Before I left for the next call he was intubated, medicated, stable, and in the operating room.

I can't help feeling great as I write this, nor do I want it to stop. Somebody is alive right now that would be dead had we not shown up with the right blend of strength and experience to do our job. To enter a blood-splattered, out-of-control scene and restore order to the madhouse while giving somebody a second chance is not something to be taken lightly. Having a capable team waiting to take over is equally important. I'm honored and privileged to be part of all this, and I thank everybody who participated in saving this patient's life.

Money Troubles

"Bodies dropping, you think it's funny. I got somethin', you wait and see, been wantin' to shoot for a while now," he said, sitting on the bed in an upstairs bedroom. He was big. Bigger than me anyway, dressed in military fatigues.

"I got somethin' for you all, what you think I can't, I been fightin' since I was ten."

"We have to take you to the hospital, your family is concerned," I said in my best, reasonable, I'm your pal voice.

"I don't need no hospital! I need to get rid of you!"

As soon as I saw him reach into the dresser I started my retreat. Graceful it was not. In my mind I always go down with the ship; in reality I'm dressed like a woman and acting like a child watching the ship sink from the safety of the life raft.

Negotiations had ceased at this point, our patient's wife and three kids waited on the first floor, hoping that by calling 911 their husband and father, who suffered with bipolar disease, would go peacefully. He had been acting strange for a few days, tonight he "went off the deep end," was making no sense and scaring the family.

"It looks like a BB gun," said Steve, standing in the way.

"And you look like an idiot," I said, pushing past him to safety.

One police officer had been upstairs, saw that the situation was going to take more manpower, and was outside radioing for help. Three officers stood at the foot of the stairs when our patient descended, walking backward, holding a handgun behind him.

For a few tense moments I watched, frozen. A man had just been shot in a confrontation with the police in North Kingston. I did not want that to happen here.

The man kept walking backwards; one of the cops quickly disarmed the man. He was fairly reasonable after that, and we took him to Rhode Island Hospital for a psychological evaluation. While en route he told us he was having some money troubles.

Language Barrier

Tommy lay on his back on an oriental rug in a home in one of the poorest sections of Providence. His mechanical wheelchair sat idle a few feet away. His mother tried to explain what happened; when she stumbled one of the guys from Engine 14 translated for her.

"He was getting off the bus like he does every day. She didn't see what happened but he started crying. The driver stopped the lift but nothing was wrong, then lowered him to the ground and she took him home. She thinks something is wrong with his left leg."

I kneeled next to him on the clean rug. What little these two had was kept immaculate.

"Does he understand?" I asked Tommy's mom. She didn't so the firefighter translated.

"He's mentally delayed, has good days and bad, usually he is very happy, never cries or complains."

I felt Tommy's legs, looking for deformities. I tried to straighten them out, then noticed the braces sitting next to his wheelchair and thought better. He was helpless, staring at me, then his mom then me again. Words between them were useless tools, their language understood by them and only them. I got a small taste when Tommy's eyes locked on mine.

He cried out when I touched his left knee. I didn't see any swelling but I just couldn't tell, and Tommy couldn't tell me. We wrapped him in a blanket and carried him outside. A bunch of kids stood at the door, eight, nine, and ten years old, and formed an honor guard as we carried their friend — or if not their friend then the kid in the wheelchair who lives on the corner—into the rescue.

We rode to the hospital in language barrier silence. Me, English with a little Spanish, her, Spanish with a little English, and Tommy with no language at all.

Except for those eyes. What goes on in his mind is a mystery to me, but I have a feeling his mom knows everything.

Afternoon Blaze

I arrived at the fire scene a minute after the first-in companies. Plenty of trucks littered the fire ground, not many firefighters. Ladder 5 was busy preparing to "get the roof," somebody was at the pump panel of Engine 10, and the chief directed the operations from Side 1. Everybody else was inside, mounting an aggressive interior attack.

It's strange being on the outside. I fought fires for ten years, seven now on the rescue. We treated three firefighters and a civilian for a variety of fire-related injuries and could have treated many more if I didn't work with a bunch of mule-headed people who don't know enough to stay down after taking a beating. The officer of Ladder 5 took a piece of roof planking to his head as I walked past him. The smoldering debris fell three floors before landing on his head.

He stumbled for a few moments, regained his balance, found his Halligan among the debris, and walked back into the fire.

Nobody listens to the rescue guy.

When Eisenhower Was President

He lives by himself in a ten-room house on Lexington Avenue. Eisenhower was president when he moved in. A lot has changed since, the tree-lined street used to be home to wealthy families, back when South Providence was *the* place to live.

"Used to be quite a place," he said to me on the way to the hospital.

"It's coming back," I answered, sounding more hopeful than I actually was.

"Never be the same."

I guess it won't. He had been vomiting since this morning, couldn't eat, was worried dehydration was setting in.

"Sorry to bother you fellas," he said while seated on the bench after walking from his home to the rescue.

"You're pretty spry for an old guy," I mentioned, impressed with his vitality. This was call number thirty since five o'clock yesterday afternoon. In that time I had carried people in their forties from their third-floor apartments because they had the flu, extricated people in their fifties from their cars after fender benders, and pretty much served as a taxi for kids with fevers. Besides a few barn burners and three or four people who actually needed us, Rescue 1 could have been Taxi 1 and nobody would have noticed.

"Well, I walk every day," he said. I imagined him walking the same streets he did when he was a young man, when Eisenhower was president.

It must break his heart, but you would never know it. I asked him about the old days during our short trip to the hospital, he willingly obliged. He was born in 1927, the same year as my father. Had he lived past sixty-one I bet he'd still be walking around the neighborhood telling me stories about the old days rather than the stranger in my truck.

Stranger or not, I'll take it. Thanks, William. And good night, Dad.

EMS1, with permission from Greg Friese, editor

Luncheon Special

Intoxicated man #1 sat quietly on the bench, appearing to doze. Heroin? Nah, just tired. The safety belt kept him upright, without it he would be on the floor. He had been sleeping peacefully next to a Dumpster before a concerned citizen with a cell phone intervened.

As usual, we were out of rescues. There must have been a luncheon special somewhere offering free half-pints of vodka to homeless people. Four out of our six rescues had been dispatched to pick up "intoxicated males."

Another call came over the radio, this time Engine 13 with a Cranston rescue. Another intoxicated male. He was on our way so we cancelled the out-of-town crew and grabbed him, a midweek two-for-one special.

Intoxicated man # 2 was sprawled out on a sidewalk. Another regular. We put him on the stretcher, keeping some distance between him and # 1. They fought with each other anyway during our ride to Rhode Island Hospital; I sat in the captain's seat filling out the paperwork, my two passengers occupied for the moment. At least they weren't fighting with me.

Ain't Lyin'

On Wednesday I brought him to the hospital. It wasn't the first, second, or fiftieth time.

"How have you been, Mo?"

"The same."

"I haven't seen you in a while."

"Been livin' with my sister."

"Beats living on the streets."

"Got that right."

I've known him for years. Can't say I like him, but he never gave me much trouble. He's a big guy, three hundred pounds at least and well over six feet. We used to pick him up from the same corner, drunk, usually, and either take him to the shelter or the hospital, depending on his level of intoxication. He's living in a three-decker for now, on the third floor with some family members. It's not a nice place, far from it. People sleep on the dirty floor, relieve themselves in the dirty bathroom, and eat in the dirty kitchen. The stairs are dark and in disrepair, sagging under my weight. Mo is a diabetic with heart problems. Most of his fifty-five years have been hard ones.

"Have you been drinking?" I asked.

"Ain't lyin', I been drinking."

"Diabetics shouldn't drink," I said. He smiled and rode to the hospital in silence.

"I hope he doesn't die up there," I said to my new partner, Adam, after we dropped Mo off. "Be a bitch getting him down."

Last night at 0330 hrs. I found out just how hard it would be. Despite our best efforts we never got a pulse, and he was pronounced dead at Rhode Island Hospital at 0417 hrs. He really died on his dirty bathroom floor at around 0325 hrs. At least he didn't die on the street.

Tired

Why are we called firefighters?

I first faced death on a cold winter afternoon in a hole twenty feet deep. An excavation job went horribly wrong, the foundation collapsed, burying the foreman. Twenty firefighters risked everything, frantically trying to dig him out. An hour later, long after the sun had set, we got him out.

One by one we climbed from the grave, happy to be alive yet sorry that we couldn't save him.

A few months later a grandmother and her baby were caught in the rear wheels of an eighteen-wheeler as it cut a corner too tightly, trying to avoid a snowbank. The baby was dragged one hundred yards in the mangled carriage, the grandmother crushed next to the snowbank. The grandmother survived, the baby did not.

Not long after a man hid in some low shrubbery, waiting for a train. When the train drew close he ran in front of it. The engineer never had a chance to slow down. The man disintegrated on impact. I walked toward the carcass, trying to avoid hundreds of quarter-sized pieces of meat, a surreal aura surrounding us as we covered what was left of the body.

With almost a year on the job I stood helplessly and watched my brother firefighters stumble from a fifteen-foot storage tank. They had been attempting to rescue a worker who was overcome by fumes while cleaning the vat and died hanging from his safety harness. Later that week I saw my friend's brother hanging in a bedroom closet. He called 911, I showed up.

By the end of my first year I had seen more than I care to remember. Between all of these calls and many more we did fight some fire. I was well into my second year when I got my first two fire victims. I remember bagging the three-year-old with one hand and doing compressions on the one-year-old until more help showed up.

Some things you never forget. I've got a lot on my mind after eighteen years, every one of those years filled with similar incidents.

Firefighters? Yeah, we're firefighters. And a whole lot more.

Why am I writing this now?

Maybe I'm a little tired of picking up the paper or turning on the news and hearing about the recent town or city that closed fire companies or reduced manning or laid firefighters off, or demanded pay cuts and benefit concessions.

Maybe I'm sick of hearing how "firefighters" shouldn't be able to shop for dinner or retire after "just twenty years."

Maybe I'm just tired.

For Whom the Bell Tolls

I've gotten used to seeing them as I drive through the neighborhoods, young guys, most of them dressed in hoodies, slow walking, slouching, nowhere to go. They are seldom alone. Yesterday one of them leaned into the side window of a parked car and put four or five bullets into a seventeen-year-old kid. Gang members? Drug dealers? Maybe. Whatever they are, they are still human beings. I still can't get over the fact that I share the same streets with people capable of pointing a gun at somebody and pulling the trigger not once or twice, but emptying the magazine into another person. There was no provocation or self-defense, just cold-blooded murder. Or attempted murder, but what difference does it make?

Rescue 1 and Engine 11 did their thing; the patient is out of surgery and in critical condition at Rhode Island Hospital. Chances are somebody else will be shot, sooner rather than later. At some point today, I probably crossed paths with people planning an execution. I'd rather not look at the world and people in it like this, but it is impossible to ignore.

Quiet now, but any minute the bell could toll.

Tense

There he sat, all four hundred pounds of him, in the middle of the street, handcuffed, shirtless, and ready to rumble. The bar crowd had already left, a few stragglers stumbled past as we lassoed the raging bull and tied him down. He snarled and spit and carried on like he was fighting for his life.

Good Guys 1

Raging Bull 0

They medicated him once we dragged him into the ER; he was still spitting and snarling when I left, though the snarling wasn't as ferocious and the spit was more like drool.

The guy on the stretcher next to him had taken a bullet to the head. As I walked out the Providence police walked another guy in handcuffs past me. The alleged shooter? So I'm told. He didn't look like somebody capable of putting a bullet into somebody's head, but what does a person capable of doing that look like? A crowd of kids converged in the parking lot and waiting room, security and police cruisers in equal numbers stood by, waiting.

Wisdom from the Mouth of Babes

I dragged myself into Rescue 5's office this morning, took the portable from Teresa, and got ready to start another shift, this time looking forward to five o'clock so I could get back to Rescue 1 and start the countdown till 0700.

Every now and then a beacon of light enters my vision, so bright it's nearly blinding. I fumble through my days, always waiting for a shift to end, a call to be over, another cycle in the books. I keep the future in mind always, at ten years I had ten to go, fifteen five more, now at eighteen two more and out, time to "enjoy my life."

"I have no idea how I'm going to be able to do this for two more years," I said to Teresa. We work the same shift, C Group, her in charge of Rescue 5, me at Rescue 1, Zack at Rescue 4, a guy who doesn't want his name in my blog at 3, and an Acting Captain at 2. We've worked together for seven or eight years now, the officers steady with a steady stream of Rescue technicians coming and going. Some of the techs stick around. Terry's partner John has been around for a while and doesn't look to be going anywhere any time soon. Can't say I blame him. Zack has Stephanie, almost a year now and holding steady. The six of us make a difficult job bearable, at times even fun.

"What if next week were your last?" asked Teresa, wanting to get home and get some rest but staying at work for a few extra minutes to talk some sense into somebody she cares about. "When you leave here you will never come back. A big part of your life will be over. Why would you want that to rush past you?"

"I don't know."

"You're not ready to leave, you love it too much. Think about your friends in the station, the hospitals, even the patients. This is an amazing ride, slow down and enjoy every minute, who knows if you'll even be alive in two years."

I don't think she is even thirty years old. I had been a firefighter for ten years when we met in EMT Cardiac class in 2000. She was just a kid who wanted to deliver babies someday. Two years later she was sworn in as a Providence firefighter. A few weeks later she was assigned to Rescue 5. A couple of weeks after that she and JoeEMT who comments here responded to Thayer Street for a man in a car who put a gun to his head and pulled the trigger. I heard the call dispatched and knew the mess they were heading toward, worried how the sight would affect her. She did okay, and continues to thrive in a field where burnout is almost a prerequisite for employment.

She even dispenses some profound advice now and then. I think she's delivered a baby or two.

Thanks, Teresa. I believe it's going to be a good day . . .

Poetic

Some of our patients are waging courageous battles against horrendous diseases. It can be easy to forget the struggles faced by so many we come in contact with. I have been linked to Susie Hemingway's poems of love for a year or so, not because I know anything about poetry, I don't. But her words make me remember why I do what I do. The following poem took my breath away.

People need us. It is a huge responsibility.

Thank you, Susie and Hamada, for making me a better firefighter, EMT, and hopefully, person.

"I Write For You"

As sun doth melt the silver days
and fresh green buds do chase away
the remnants of these chilly days,
I write for you . . .
you sleep and sleep my only love
you miss spring birds and clouds above,
in dreaming slumber, days do pass, and
even though against the breeze
the fragile words do come to me,
still sleep stays on those lovely eyes,
for days are shorter dear for you
the circle smaller, in violet blue,
again the sun will find its rays
to warm your heart and fill your days
and I will spend my time with you
in quiet gentle solitude,
till this day, my only love,
I write for you . . .
soon once again, dear God for me
you'll sit on swing, beneath the trees,
to listen to the buzzing bees

the rustle of the summer leaves,
then you will snuggle close to me,
when smudges of my tears
do fall, to stain the ink,
and you will sleep,
and I will write
my words for thee . . .

Susie Hemingway

What's In a Name?

She fell from her bed onto a carpeted floor, no obvious injury, cried immediately, and then laughed. Her mom just "wanted her checked." The responsibility that people thrust upon me is a bit too much at times, so I did what any self-respecting EMT would do — thrust the responsibility onto somebody else. Off we went to Hasbro Children's Hospital.

It was a relatively long ride to the hospital, at least by Providence standards. Most of my transports can be done in less than ten minutes, a lot of them in less than five. This one took almost fifteen. I wish it took longer.

My patient, securely snuggled in her car seat that I had attached to the stretcher, captivated me right from the start. She looked me in the eye as we got moving and didn't look away.

"She's beautiful," I said, looking up as I started my report.

"Her father is Intuit Indian, I'm half Egyptian and half Puerto Rican," said the proud mama.

An Egyptian Eskimo from Puerto Rico, right here in Providence, RI.

"What is her name?" I asked Mom.

"Karizma."

"No way."

"Yup. I just liked the way it sounds, like it fit her."

"It does."

"Her middle name is charming."

"What is it?" I asked.

"Charming."

"I know, what . . . never mind."

With a first name like Karizma, could Charming be far behind?

"Karizma Charming Morales."

Perfect.

Family

"Engine 10 to Rescue 1, eighty-year-old female, respiratory distress, possible CHF."

"Rescue 1, received."

We turned the corner onto a narrow dead end street just off of Broad. The door of the last house on the left was open, frenzied activity just beyond the threshold.

"Get the chair," I said to Adam and entered the home.

"230/115, pulsox 68 percent," said Ted as I approached the patient. She was struggling to breathe, her lungs full of fluid. The oxygen mask covered the bottom half of her face, her eyes were panicked. Adam set the chair up next to her, the guys from Engine 10 picked her from the couch and got her ready to move. Seven or eight family members stood nearby, some worried, some afraid, some near panic.

"What is her name?" I asked.

"Auriela," one of the women answered.

I took a nitro from the bottle I had put in my pocket and had the woman tell Auriela to put it under her tongue and let it melt. She struggled for a while, then understood. A minute later we were in the rescue, Ted applying EKG leads, Adam starting an IV, and myself preparing an albuterol treatment.

"I'll give you a driver and an extra set of hands in back," Frank, the officer of Engine 10, said, closing the rear doors of the rescue.

"Let's roll."

We began our journey toward Rhode Island Hospital, three of us in the back with the patient, a firefighter from Engine 10 driving the rescue, and Frank and Paul following with the engine. Another nitro en route, 40 ml of Lasix and the albuterol treatment seemed to be effective; Auriela's eyes stopped darting, her breathing slowed as her lungs cleared, and she actually managed a little smile. The frantic activity in the back of the rescue slowed in rhythm with our patient's breathing. There wasn't much more to do but comfort her, let her know she would be all right. She didn't speak a word of English, and we barely spoke a word of Spanish, but all of us knew she was out of the woods.

We arrived at the hospital. The rear doors of the rescue opened and there stood one of our guys, an off-duty firefighter from Engine 11. I looked at him for a moment, confused.

"That's my grandmother," he said, helping us wheel her in.

Twenty minutes later he shook my hand as we were preparing to leave.

"Thanks, Mike, you guys were incredi..."

I can't imagine a more satisfying job than the one I have.

Founding Fathers

Every day I'm forced to cat... segment of our society who do nothing to contribu... One of the many inspiring in the history of civiliz... ability to protect those who things about Americ... Our collective charity defines cannot protect the... world conquest and domination yet us; a people cap... within our borders, create wealth, content to sta...

produce food bountiful enough to feed the world, and live our lives as productive protectors of freedom. The cost is staggering. Our many societal ills could be eradicated if we chose to close our borders and take care of our own.

Instead, we choose to let our own take care of themselves, the philosophy that we all have a right to pursue happiness proven more effective than happiness being provided to us by a collective system of wealth distribution. We struggle. We go hungry. We want. A healthy fear keeps us motivated; failure is not an option. Or is it?

I see a population beaten by promises made by modern-day politicians who tell their constituents that they "deserve" everything we now consider necessities, not because they have earned it, rather because they live here, as though merely populating a land mass made great by those who have sacrificed, starved, and died to provide it is enough.

Well, folks, existing is not enough. Giving to people who expect the charity of others as their right and privilege is not enough. Eventually the givers get tired of giving to those not worthy of their charity. Resentment grows as pockets empty. It is impossible for a person to stay productive for the benefit of another. We have reached the tipping point. Many have given up, and aspire only to stay below a mandated level of success, thus entitling themselves to the "generosity" of the government. To rise above the poverty level means giving up free healthcare, subsidized housing, and many more benefits keeping people poor and powerless.

Nobody deserves free healthcare. Nobody deserves prosperity. Nobody deserves free anything other than what they have earned. Our generosity has failed. Miserably. This is not the country I wish to live in its present state.

I'll go on providing free emergency rooms for people who lack the gumption emergency rooms for provided by the working taxpayers on a free service this nation. I'll listen to them explain how they called 911 so they could access free medical care faster. I'll deliver them to the places that will give them their antibiotics for their sniffles, or take fifteen-year-old children to maternity wards so they can deliver their babies into a world of benefits.

I'll do it because every now and then somebody truly needs help, and I'll be damned if I'll turn my back on somebody in need. Real need.

Wrong Way
4:00 a.m. I'm driving down 95 South toward an MVA on 95 North. Originally we were sent to Exit 19, nothing there, I radioed dispatch.

"Rescue 1 to fire alarm, 95 North is clear to the 195 split, any more information?"

"Stand by, Rescue 1, we have a report the accident is at Exit 16."

Received, turning around.

Six minutes had passed since the original dispatch.

"Fire alarm to Rescue 1 and Engine 13, we're sending Engine 11 to cover the northbound lanes."

"Roger."

Two more minutes passed.

"Engine 11 to fire alarm." Miles, sounding like he was ordering a pizza, as usual. *"We've got a pedestrian struck, female in her twenties, have Rescue 1 step it up."*

I looked over to the northbound lanes at the scene, a hundred feet away seeming like a hundred miles. A car was in the breakdown lane, emergency lights flashing. Twenty feet in front of the car was a person covered with a sheet.

"Rescue 1, received." I put the mic back in the cradle and did an inventory. The wife, home in bed, the kids, hopefully home in bed, everybody else I know's kids, I couldn't think about it. Bottom line, some poor soul's kid was lying on 95 covered with a sheet. And I was heading south, waiting for the exit where I could turn it around, nothing to do but wait.

I can't think of a worse image than a person covered with a sheet, lying on Interstate 95 at four in the morning and a rescue heading in the opposite direction.

Adam did a great job getting us there in three minutes, should have taken four or five; I wasn't paying attention, just clearing my mind.

We stopped the rescue next to the victim. The crew from Engine 11 had an IV started, collar in place and ready to go. The girl, twenty-five years old, was still conscious. Her friend had run out of gas, she was putting a gallon in when a car sideswiped her. Luckily, it didn't hit full force; the impact spun her around, threw her ten or so feet in the air, and she landed twenty feet away.

We did our thing, immobilized, IV O2, EKG and trauma assessment and got her to the hospital five minutes after our arrival. As we left the scene we passed a bright green highway sign, EXIT 19, 2 MILES. The original caller must have seen that sign and given the wrong location.

The patient was in Trauma 3 when I left, her friend who had run out of gas waiting outside.

It looks like she's going to make it.

Records

She opened her door a crack and peered from the darkness, letting a cloud of smoke escape from her tiny apartment. She's fifty-four, lives alone, and listens to forty-year-old records on an old turntable. She spends her days drinking and living in the past, her and her memories. I think she was pretty once.

"What do you have, Cheech and Chong hiding in there?" I asked, waving the smoke away.

"I'm not going to Rhode Island Hospital."

"Really."

"They don't know what they're doing."

"Yes they do."

"I'm not going anywhere. Just leave me alone!"

I put my foot in front of the door before she could close it. It bounced back on her. She backed up and sat on her bed.

"I'm sick and you don't care."

"Really."

"Nobody cares, I want to die!"

"Oh, come on now, if you wanted to die you wouldn't have called us."

"My belly hurts! I have pancreatitis!"

"Then why did you drink?"

"Because I'm in pain!"

"You're in pain because you drank."

"Go away."

"You're coming with me."

"Not if we're going to Rhode Island."

"Rhode Island is the closest hospital; if you were looking for a ride you should have called a taxi."

"I knew you didn't care!"

"Oh, stop it, we'll take you to Miriam Hospital."

"I'm not going anywhere!"

She leapt from the bed and tried again to slam the door. Again it struck my foot and bounced back on her.

"That's it, I'm leaving. If you want to, come meet me in the truck."

I closed the door behind me and retreated to the rescue. Before I made it my patient ran past me, opened the rear doors, and threw herself onto the stretcher.

"The blood pressure cuff is next to you, do you mind getting your own vitals?"

She crossed her arms and didn't speak again until we arrived at Miriam. There, she informed the charge nurse that she was leaving, and asked me if I would give her a ride home.

At first the people at Miriam were going to let her go. I advised them of her history and probable alcohol use, they decided she had better stay. They put her on a stretcher in the hallway, all the rooms were full.

She didn't want to be there, and they didn't want her. I think she has a long wait in front of her, and she doesn't have her records to keep her company.

Police and Thieves

2300 hrs. An hour till midnight. Desperate man breaks into bakery.

2311 hrs. Desperate man spotted by concerned citizen.

2318 hrs. Police arrive.

2319 hrs. Desperate man steals van, chase ensues.

2330 hrs. Chase ends on Rt. 195.

2331 hrs. Desperate man jumps twenty-five feet from Rt. 195 onto grassy knoll, rolls over and runs into the Providence River.

2336 hrs. Providence Police drag desperate man from riverbank.

2339 hrs. Rescue 5 and Engine 9 dispatched for "a man in the water."

2343 hrs. PFD on scene.

2344 hrs. Desperate man treated, hypothermia, poss ankle fracture, poss spinal injury.

2348 hrs. Desperate man transported to RIH ER.

2355 hrs. Desperate man sedated.

0015 hrs. Rescue 5 in quarters and off.

Any excuse to get the Clash on my mind will do. I was a high school sophomore when "Police and Thieves" was released. To this day, whenever I hear The Clash it's like my first time. I can't think of anything else that feels as good.

Well, maybe one other thing but I was a high school senior when I found that!

Happy Endings?

Prostitution is legal in Providence. Asian spas have blossomed everywhere, offering "sensual massage." Every now and then the media does a story on the people behind the facade, subsequently the politicians make a little noise, then it all goes away.

It never goes away for the people providing the service. I've read accounts of young Asian women and girls lured from their homes with promises of a better life here in America, only to find themselves indebted to their supposed benefactors.

Little is known about this segment of our society. The very nature of the business assures discretion. I've often wondered about the people involved in this life. Are they involved in some lurid sex slave ring, or are they merely providing a service with willing employees making a living at the oldest profession we know?

Man Down

"Why are you two laying on top of each other?"

"We went man down."

"You went what?"

"Man down. Call 911."

"You look like homosexuals."

That got their attention. One crawled off the other; they dusted the mulch off their filthy clothes and tried to stand. One succeeded, the other stayed "man down."

"We not fags, man, we ain't Will and Grace."

"Who?"

"You know who. Bellhopper and the Fridge."

"They're gay?"

"Ya think?"

Bellhopper and the Fridge are two homeless guys who have prowled these streets for years. At one time they were loners; recently when one calls the other isn't far behind. Whichever one is more coherent makes sure the other is taken care of. It never occurred to me they might be more than friends. The fact that they have usually pissed and shit themselves before somebody called 911 to clean them off the streets probably has something to do with it. I just can't imagine them having the capacity for sexual relations, gay or not.

"You guys keep going 'man down' and they'll be calling you Will and Grace."

"We ain't no Will and Grace! We like the poossy!"

The one who briefly stood fell back into the bushes, next to his buddy. We fished them out and took them in.

Resurrection

Eyes closed, barely breathing, track marks up his arms. Family stands by, nervously laughing, trying to act nonchalant. Face purple now as a needle of a different sort enters his arm. Glass vial shines, reflected light from the overhead. Underwear soaked, ice cubes roll around the floor, picking up pubic hair when they near the shower. I crouch next to him, less contact with the floor the better. Breathing slow, two a minute, oxygen nearby, bag valve mask ready. Quiet now as the Narcan enters his bloodstream. Minute passed. Eyes flutter. Purple turns to red, to grey, to white. Eyes open. Breathing normal. Family sighs and moves on. Stretcher comes to bathroom door. A sheet appears, covers him. IV ripped from arm, restraints placed. Into the night, a man in his underwear, recently resurrected, enters the rescue. The doors close.

Go Home

She's twenty-four and homeless, and has been for four years. She has kids back in Ohio, had to leave them there when it was time to find a better life for herself. She found Rhode Island. At nine o'clock at night she wandered into Kennedy Plaza, the main bus station in Providence, and slumped against a wall. A police officer told her to move on, she said she couldn't. The police called us.

"What's the matter?"

"I can't move."

"You can't move."

"I've been walking all day and can't walk anymore."

"Get in the truck."

I've given up. I used to fight to maintain some resemblance of dignity concerning EMS and the 911 system; now I operate as if I'm part social services agency, part homeless advocate, rolling medicine cabinet, part taxi, and occasional emergency medical technician.

She managed to move, this time ambling into the rescue. She slowly stepped in and sat on the bench seat. I sat across from her, Adam drove toward Rhode Island Hospital where the cure for "inability to move" waited.

"Why have you been walking all day?"

"I have nowhere to go. I'm homeless."

"Where are you from?"

"Akron, Ohio."

"Why don't you go back?"

"They only have one homeless shelter in the state! They don't have no food kitchens, nothin'! I can't even get a coffee!"

"Why did you come here?"

"Three hots and a cot. Everybody knows this is a good place. Every day of the week somebody's got somethin'. Sundays at the Amos House, every day at the McCauley

House, soup kitchens, shelters, people give you money just for holding up a sign."

"Why don't you go to Tent City?" referring to a notorious homeless encampment under an I-195 bridge in Providence.

"They threw me out."

"You got thrown out of Tent City? Why?"

"I didn't play by their rules."

Rules? I didn't know there were any rules. We arrived at the hospital. I walked my patient in. A young girl from Ohio living on the streets of Providence, getting by mainly from the generosity of others. Our generosity is harming her more than helping her. She would be better off in Akron, learning how to be responsible and taking care of her children.

The Garden
The basement was cold, musty, and when alone a little scary. A space heater hissed and crackled, hot to the touch, ugly yet comforting. Asbestos tile covered the floor, doors on one side of the room opened to a narrow passageway where the heart of the home sat, called upon to provide warmth when needed, forgotten when not. The "Christmas Stuff" waited in the little closet under the stairs, now and then a little smell of Christmas would escape between the louvers of the door, spreading more warmth into "the Garden."

A couch sat in front of an old RCA television console, reserved for game night. Wires snaked from the back of the cabinet, stapled against the paneled walls, into the passageway and out the cellar window, up the side of the house next to the chimney and onto the roof. The latest in television technology was planted there, much like the American flag was planted on the surface of the moon earlier that summer, only this was no flag, it was a rotary antenna.

Some nights the picture was almost clear when the antenna pointed north, toward Boston. Sometimes turning it northeast worked better, and for some mysterious reason pointing it south provided the best picture on the weekends. Even the best picture was always obscured by "snow." It never occurred to us that some day we might actually see the puck.

If there is heaven on earth, it was in the basement of 19 Haley Road on Game Night.

My father watched nearly every game on that old TV, inviting his fan club to his lair where we would make it through the first period, slumber during the second, and be out cold by the third. Occasionally a thrown empty would crash against the TV screen, the anger directed at some hooligan from the other team, usually a Canadian, but the bums on the Rangers weren't much better. If the noise woke us, we might see the end of the game before sneaking up the stairs to bed.

The year before he died my wife and I took my father to Boston Garden for a Bruins game. The old place was scheduled to be torn down soon, we were afraid we were running out of time. Turns out we were, but not for the reason we expected.

He had followed the team since the thirties and never set foot on the hallowed ground. It was a magical moment when he entered the arena, stopped in his tracks as he looked toward the ghost-filled rafters and saw firsthand the championship banners that had collected over the decades. It was if the earth stood still. He stood, hypnotized, tears filling his eyes but not escaping; never escaping, and took it all in. For a man who started following his team by listening to the "Original Six" on the radio, it was a near perfect moment.

For his son who spent the best years of his childhood in a magical basement, it was.

Mutual Admiration Society

The latest meeting of the mutual admiration society was in full swing as we drove through the East Side. Adam and I talked about how fabulous we were, knowledgeable, dashing lifesavers with no peers, here or anywhere. Why we had to share the same earth with lesser beings escaped us as we cruised Thayer Street, looking for a cup of coffee worthy of such brilliant EMTs.

The previous job went off without a hitch, a fifty-nine-year-old female found slumped at her desk, a call made to 911, rapid response by the closest fire company, we arrived from the opposite end of the city in eight minutes.

She had reported for work, said hello to coworkers, poured herself a cup of coffee, and walked to her office. A friend found her a short time later, slumped and semiconscious. Our exam showed left-side weakness with facial droop, hypertensive and confused. Possible CVA.

As her coworkers and various onlookers watched, oxygen was administered, the patient extricated from her basement office, history obtained, IV established, vitals assessed, hospital notified, and the patient transported within fifteen minutes of dispatch, approximately thirty minutes from onset of symptoms.

Every now and then a call goes perfectly, the patient given prompt, efficient treatment with a hopefully positive outcome, and the onlookers and friends fall over each other trying to touch us as we leave, or even share the same space, hoping some of what we have might rub off on them. We casually bask in the glory, accept the accolades as our right and privilege, and wait for the next cry for help from the citizenry we are sworn to protect.

A sixty-year-old man has fallen and struck his head on a tile floor. We respond. Wrong straps on the backboard, wrong size cervical collar, and proceed to go downhill from there.

We finally secure the patient to the backboard and place him backwards on the stretcher as the collar that is supposed to be providing c-spine immobilization moves from under the patient's chin and begins to suffocate him. He violently shakes his head back and forth, freeing himself from his restraint, and verbally attacks his rescuers. Our capes firmly stuffed between our legs, we try to right the situation as we explain that his feet are at the head of the stretcher and his head is at the feet.

Somehow we get him to the rescue without paralyzing him, lift him inside, and botch three IV attempts. Add mangled arm to his list of injuries. An air leak has rendered the truck's suspension useless, it feels as if we're riding a hay wagon down a rocky trail on our way to the hospital. What began as a head laceration with no loss of consciousness is now a level 1 trauma.

Our patient somehow survives his ordeal, his coworkers and family wait for us at the ER, forming a gauntlet as we wheel their loved one past them. I swear some are holding pitchforks and torches. Our heroes pass the patient over to the ER staff, then slink out of the hospital, avoiding eye contact with the angry mob that has formed.

Another call for help comes in as we call to a close the latest meeting of the mutual admiration society. Good thing there were only two members.

EMS World

Twilight
Noon. Hour nineteen of thirty-eight. Sixteen calls so far, long way to go. Me and Adam are riding back to the station.

"The sun is hurting my eyes."

"That's because you lost your sunglasses."

"I think something far more sinister is going on."

Flashback—seven hours ago . . .

0523 hrs. Predawn. Dispatched to a tenement house in South Providence for a suicidal pregnant twenty-year-old with arm lacerations. I stand on the third-floor landing listening to Oliver talk to the girl and her boyfriend. I can't get up the rest of the stairs, all forward progress has stopped, the guys from Engine 10 and two Providence police officers clog the narrow, dimly lit stairway. I'm quite happy to wait at the end of the line and listen.

"Did you try to hurt yourself?" asks Oliver.

"She cut her wrist with a broken crack pipe," comes a male voice from above.

"Were you smoking crack?"

"Not us, she's pregnant."

The line turns toward me and heads down the stairs. I lead the march into the street and toward the rescue. A pretty, pale woman joins me in back.

"I'm all set," I say to the cops and firefighters, Adam goes in front to drive. My patient's cuts are superficial, scratches really. She stares intently at me as I begin my report.

"What happened?"

"He was going to hurt me," she states in a regal manner, very articulate. "He planned to cut me and drink my blood."

I look over the edge of the paper and see her eyes focused intently on mine, not blinking, not moving, as if I'm prey.

"Why did he want to do that?"

"I stopped him by cutting myself," she replies, ignoring my question, still staring. I'm a little unnerved. She has an old-fashioned way of speaking, as if she has been alive for centuries. Her skin is even more pale in the dim light of the rescue, translucent. Her eyes are bloodshot, but intense. I can't wait to get to the hospital. Thankfully the rescue slows, turns, and backs into the rescue bay. I quickly stand and help my patient out the door. She clutches my arm with her wounded one, some blood is transferred.

"Thank you, you've been very kind." I wouldn't say she smiled, but her face showed amusement, as if we're in on something together. She continued to stare, and as I left I looked over my shoulder and she still stared, still amused.

0730 hrs. Dispatched to a methadone clinic for a man who can't walk. I uncross my arms from the front of my chest, open my eyes, and rise from my slumber. It's warm, the sun hurts my skin. I roll down my sleeves and squint into the glaring sun. A small man, troll-like, stands at the bottom of the hill at the entrance to the clinic. He stares as we pass. I walk inside the clinic and ask who called 911, nobody answers. The troll runs up the hill, stands in front of the rescue, and tells me he can't walk.

"You just ran up the hill."

"I can't get on the bus."

"But you can run up a hill?"

The troll goes bananas, starts taking off his clothes to show me his MRSA scars, his deformities, and tells me he is HIV+ with hepatitis C.

"I need to go to the hospital."

"Get in."

I'm tired. The troll is annoying. I can't understand a word he is saying as he rants and raves all the way to the hospital, less than one mile away. His language is foreign, possibly Latin. I swear his head turned 360 degrees when I looked away. He stares at me after we drop him off at the hospital and doesn't look away. The stare stays with me all the way back to the station. I enter my office, turn out the light, and close the shades. The sun still hurts. I can't wait till night.

Three calls come and go with nothing strange happening. I think I'll be okay.

1436 hrs. Called to a high-rise for a man with chest pains. Adam gets in the truck and starts it. I say something, he jumps, startled, and says he didn't see me sitting there. Interesting,

I'll have to find a mirror and see if there is a reflection. We arrive and find a seventy-two-year-old Haitian man with a dried chicken claw tied around his neck, hung on a loose rawhide cord.

"Are you a voodoo priest?" I ask.

"Yes," he replies. "And, I'm the son of Satan." He also has hep C and HIV.

I swear I'm not making this up.

As the call progresses and I treat the son of Satan, who also happens to be having chest pain with ST elevations, I find him to be quite pleasant. He is deathly afraid of needles, but tells me I have a gift as I sink one into his arm. The blood is rich and red as it drips from his arm onto the 4 × 4. It is fascinating, this blood, I think to myself as I finish up the IV, give him some aspirin and nitro, and ride together to the hospital. He shakes my hand and stares into my eyes as I'm about to leave. I have a difficult time looking away.

Five more calls, nothing strange. If a Catholic priest calls 911 tonight I'll start to worry.

Darkness descends. I'm in my office, waiting for the night to begin. It's the first warm Friday night of the season. Should be a bloodbath.

Spots

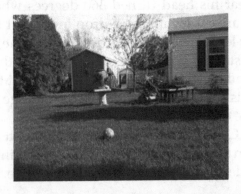

It occurred to me as I was cutting the grass that brown spots, holes, and prison breaks weren't all that bad.

On a happier note, I turned forty-seven today. I always thought forty-seven was old, and I guess it is, but in the words of the immortal Ronnie Van Zant from Lynyrd Skynyrd during a break at one of his shows in the seventies, after rocking the house for over two hours, "Hell, I ain't even worked up a sweat yet!"

Instinct

Baby in one hand, railing in the other. She takes the first step down toward the basement; the railing pulls from the wall. Mom loses balance and begins to fall. She somehow manages to maneuver her body so that her back bears the brunt of the fall, possibly breaking a rib or two when she hits the cement steps. The baby is blissfully unaware and rests comfortably while her mother bounces down seven stairs.

She is in excruciating pain when we arrive. She managed to make her way to the top of the stairs where she sat, sobbing. Not much more than a baby herself, her instinct took over at the moment of truth. Extrication is a little more bearable for her thanks to some pain management steps made prior to movement. All she cared about was if her baby was okay.

Happy Early Mother's Day.

Supplemental Budget
For Immediate Release

Michael Morse submitted his plan to close a $200 weekly deficit, and with it comes a clear-cut picture of how the plan will work.

In a completely ignored news conference Monday morning on the front steps of his home, Morse focused on his proposed healthcare changes and five-year wage freeze, as well as his underfunded pension and lack of Social Security benefits.

Every person currently doing business with Morse is being asked to participate in his plan to balance his budget by the end of fiscal year 2010.

For example, Morse plans to stop paying co-pays for prescription drugs and doctors visits, and cutting his $100 emergency room payment in half with a projected annual savings of $2,600. These fees are simply unsustainable. Supermarkets are being asked to lower their prices until this economic crisis passes, realizing an additional $1,380 in annual savings. Waitstaff in area restaurants will no longer receive the customary 15 percent tip, 8 percent will now be the norm.

Morse will defer payments to the Warwick Sewer Authority pending a decision in small claims court regarding a fire hydrant currently occupying space on his property. Morse has long maintained that water is ridiculously expensive; the judge's ruling should absolve him of any payments exceeding $500, realizing an additional $700 in yearly savings.

All work performed at Morse's house will be subject to a 20 percent co-pay by the person doing the work. Plumbers, electricians, and all other contract labor will adhere to these new cost-saving measures until the economic crisis passes. This plan will save the Morse budget in two ways: The contractor will charge less for work performed because their co-pay will also be less. And appliance repairmen with their gold-plated service call fees will no longer be tolerated; a set hourly fee will be paid.

Charitable contributions will cease immediately. Also, all pets will be asked to leave. These pets will not be replaced until the current economic crisis passes.

The plan calls for full participation by all. If Morse can achieve concessions this year, his financial crisis will be averted, placing him in a better position for 2011.

Denial

A middle-aged man in an old man's body shuffles into the back of the rescue, groans, then sits heavily on the bench. I follow and take my seat in the captain's chair. He's fifty-three, looks seventy-five, and has been vomiting blood for two days. This isn't the first time I've taken him in for similar problems, but it may be the last. He's about done.

"You have to stop drinking."

"I been good for two months, just a couple a day."

"That's too many, you have cirrhosis of the liver."

"My doctor said I could have a drink now and then."

"When was that, 1968?"

He looks away, first out the rear window then at the floor. His vitals are stable. Amazing how little vital signs actually tell us, because he is dying. I look at him as we ride in silence toward the emergency room, knowing that within a month or two he will be dead. For now he maintains that strange, fearless optimism, thinking he can go on drinking forever, as if the party will never stop. His body has quit, the mind never really got going.

Good luck, David, I say to him as we leave the hospital. He nods and looks around the ER, looking for somebody to talk to.

Explosion

I left the station last night around five thirty, couldn't wait to get out and leave the city behind. While I was at home, sound asleep, an explosion rocked the south side of the city, a few miles away. Engine 13 and Rescue 1 were dispatched to Ocean and Pavilion for a report of a car into a house. When they arrived the car was empty but had compromised a gas meter, the smell of gas strong. A police officer stood nearby as the crews from Rescue 1 and Engine 13 began operations. The gas leak needed to be stopped, victims accounted for. A few seconds later the explosion threw the firefighters and police officer into the street, covering them with debris. Two are still hospitalized, a cop and a firefighter. The other guys are okay for now; I've talked to a few of them, they sound shell-shocked. To be honest, I'm a little shell-shocked. We joke with one another all the time, "It's all fun and games until somebody loses an eye," things like that. Now and then one of us gets hurt, twisted ankles, cuts and bruises, an occasional broken bone; all things that will heal. Less often but not less often enough somebody gets it badly and doesn't return.

I'm going to make it a point to hang around at shift change, at least for a couple of minutes, and catch up with people I sometimes take for granted. The guys from B Group are mostly from my training academy, the 42nd. In a few weeks or months they'll be back, picking right up where they left off, a few more scars to add to the collection.

Get well, B Group, see you soon.

Brothers from Another Mother
All present and accounted for. I took Keith home from Rhode Island Hospital tonight. He took the brunt of the explosion, according to witnesses was thrown thirty feet, suffered a concussion, lots of stitches to his head and hand and some bumps and bruises. Not bad for a guy who's on the other side of fifty. Talked to the other guys, they're home recuperating, their presence with their families the best Mother's Day present anybody could ask for.

The police officer that was injured as badly as Keith said he saw "bodies flying," and wouldn't rest until he found out if "the firemen" were all right. He ended up in the same room as Keith. Public safety organizations are like a big family, cops and firemen sometimes seem like distant cousins. Not tonight.

Get well, brothers.

The Fox

I took a walk today, slow at first, then faster until I was almost running. Then I was running, not a graceful sprint by any means, just arms and legs pumping, my heart racing, feeling good just to be alive and well. The neighborhood where I now live is like a park where people put homes. Different trees sprouting different flowers, the ground erupting with different colors every day, the grass, freshly cut this weekend, glistens with moisture from an early morning shower, only now the sun has appeared, and with the warmth the water evaporates, giving the air a freshly showered feel.

No cars today, most people are at work. Just me, the birds, and an occasional dog walker. When I think my heart is ready to explode I slow down and stroll the last half mile, just enjoying the sounds around me. A fox sprints away from my bird feeder as I walk up my driveway. He looks a little old, grey around the whiskers and not as fast as you might think a fox would be. My neighbor who knows everything told me that foxes are not necessarily nocturnal, so rabies probably isn't a factor. Too bad Mr. Fox didn't hang around, we could have had breakfast together.

I've been told my grandfather had a pet fox named Reginald. Maybe I'll catch this guy and keep him.

Nah, I'll just let him be.

Elementary

"Dr. Watson," I addressed my companion, "we have an elderly male lying on the floor in his rent-subsidized apartment, dressed only in his blue, sailboat-patterned pajama bottoms."

I took a puff from my pipe and scanned the room.

"Numerous large prescription bottles on the kitchen table lead me to believe this man has multiple medical problems."

I tapped the pipe on the kitchen table, lit a match, and reignited the pungent tobacco, disguising the stale aroma of urine.

"The television is tuned to the Spanish Channel. I must surmise that this man speaks no English, thus the dull look when I asked him his name."

"Inspector!" Watson looked up from the patient, alarmed. "See here. A scar runs down the middle of his chest!"

"Elementary, my dear Watson," I said, stepping toward the prone patient. "Look closely. The scar is neatly formed, perfectly placed, and exactly six inches in length. This is no diabolical organ thievery; this man has had open heart surgery!"

"Of course! That explains . . . nothing really. Why is he lying on the floor?"

I crouched lower, touching the patient, looking for more clues. His skin was cool and clammy. I gently shook him, he only moaned in response. Using my penlight I looked deep into his eyes. The pupils responded.

"Dr. Watson, prepare a field glucose test. We need more information!"

As Watson drew a small droplet of blood from the mysterious man's finger I looked for more clues, first assessing his vital signs, then giving him some supplemental oxygen.

"Inspector! His glucose level is dangerously low!"

"Of course it is, my good man. Prepare to solve the case!"

Now that the mystery was nearly solved, other clues became apparent. Diabetic medication was mixed with cardiac pills. A glass of orange juice, spilled next to the patient, an open and empty sugar package nearby.

Dr. Watson prepared an IV while I drew up some medication. We pushed the D-50 into the mystery man's veins and waited. A minute passed. Slowly, his eyelids began to flutter.

"I believe we are well on our way, Doctor!" I said, exhaling a cloud of smoke into the cramped apartment. "Well done!"

The patient regained consciousness, sat up, and looked around. He spoke no English but was oriented.

"We have to take him in for questioning," I said as we cleaned up the scene. We helped him onto our stretcher and locked the door behind us as we left.

Another mystery solved, in a city full of them. Not long after, we sat in my den on Baker Street ruminating. I swirled my brandy and watched the amber liquid briefly cling to the snifter's glass before reforming at the bottom.

"Cheers, Dr. Watson," I said as the glasses in our hands met with the sound that has warmed many a celebration throughout the centuries.

I drained the snifter as Watson sipped, and we sat amicably whilst waiting for the next one.

It never takes long . . .

In My Hands

The pill bottle was sticky and a little moist. I returned it to the shopping bag and peered in. There it was. The clear vial, possibly a spice container in another life, lay on its side, the contents smaller now, stuck to the bottom of the vial. The bag smelled faintly of cloves, maybe residue from before.

I looked at my hand, the fingertips glistening from the contact with the vial. I sat there and watched my hand in the dim fluorescent light as the rescue sped toward Women and Infants Hospital, a few miles away. I moved my fingers, still mesmerized. My stomach rolled, a little vomit tried to make its way from the bottom of my stomach. I forced it down. The vial of hand sanitizer was just out of reach, over near the heart monitor. I leaned on the back of the stretcher and grabbed it, pumping ten or twelve times, filling my palm with the antiseptic lotion, then rubbed my hands together as we rode in silence.

My patient was stable for now, crying softly to herself in the stretcher as one of her sons looked on. He came with us to act as an interpreter, only no words needed to be said. He just looked at his mom, then the floor, then shyly at me, then the floor again. I dried my hands on a towel, wiped the back of the stretcher, and closed my eyes.

The truck stopped. The sobbing did not. The patient's other son, husband, and ten-year-old daughter waited for us outside the rescue, greeting us when I opened the rear door. Only the ten-year-old smiled. She put her hand on the stretcher as we wheeled her mom in.

The nurse working triage asked what we had. I explained the story to her quietly, trying to keep the confidentiality intact.

"We were called for a woman having abdominal pain following an abortion, arrived to find her lying on the couch. On the kitchen table were these." I opened the bag and showed her. "Inside the clear bottle are the results of a miscarriage. There was some fluid in the vial but it spilled inside the bag."

The nurse looked at the blob of tissue drying in the bottom of the bottle. It had resembled a fetus prior to spilling in the bag and onto my hands. She closed the bag, signed my report, and took the patient in the back. I washed my hands and said goodbye to the family.

Affirmative Action

We've been hiring more minorities lately, something I'm always uneasy about. I know a lot of people who have taken the firefighter exam, done quite well after months or years of preparation, and then watched their dreams fizzle as affirmative action takes over.

I've also responded to calls with the first black female firefighter in Providence and seen the eyes of the little girls in the projects light up when they see her, possibly seeing for the first time that yes, anything truly *is* possible.

My friend and partner from a few years ago, Renato, can walk into any neighborhood in this city, talk the talk, and find out what exactly is wrong, all while setting a fine example for some of the possibly troubled Hispanic kids that hang around these streets.

The other day I was sent on a call with "Tang," an Asian, tattooed monster of a man with a heart of gold and disposition of a comedian for a combative, out-of-control twelve-year-old who had defecated on the school gym floor and eaten it. We walked past a gauntlet of schoolteachers, psychiatrists, police officers, and the vice principal toward our patient. I let Tang take the lead, he scares me, figured the kid would be petrified. Tang took a look at the patient, wrinkled his nose, and simply asked, "Did you wipe your butt?"

The kid shook his head no, stood up, and walked with my partner out to the rescue, through the throng of people who just couldn't reach him. We took the little guy to the hospital (he never did eat his shit), where Tang led him to the restroom and waited outside while he cleaned himself up. I'm sure the kid has serious emotional problems and will act out again, but for now, that moment he found peace and understanding from a guy who looked like he just got released from prison.

Do I believe in affirmative action? I honestly don't know anymore.

Priceless

Her water broke as she stepped into the rescue. She lay on the stretcher and said, "I think I'm having the baby."

"What is your due date?"

"June 15."

I relaxed, secure in my knowledge that modern medical technology is never wrong about these things. If they say the due date is the fifteenth, the fifteenth it shall be.

"Don't worry, you're not due for a while. We'll get you to the hospital in plenty of time."

"I really think I'm having the baby."

I covered her with a sheet and had a look-see. All quiet on the southern front. Just to be safe we took a driver from Engine 8 and one of their guys in back and started the six-minute trek to Women and Infants Hospital.

"Are there any complications?" I asked the forty-year-old woman whose second child seemed intent on making an early entry into this world.

"I really think I'm having this baby now."

I lifted the sheet and took another look. That wasn't there a minute ago.

"Rick, you may want to step it up," I said to the driver as we approached the I-95 on-ramp, looking away for a moment.

I took another look.

"I think you're having the baby."

Rescue ride to Women and Infants, $450.

Supplemental oxygen, $25.

Umbilical clamps, $13.

The look on the mother's face when I repeated her words . . . priceless.

I placed the palm of my right hand gently on the crowning head and felt mom's abdomen. For some unknown reason I rubbed her belly like a genie lamp, slow circular motions.

"You know, having a baby in a moving rescue isn't all that bad," I said, or something equally ridiculous as I continued rubbing her belly. She shouted, just a little. I looked down.

Mark and Adam had the emergency maternity kit open, clamps lined up, scalpel ready, blanket open, bulb syringe ready, pedi mask standing by.

Three minutes away from my salvation. If she could only hold on.

Instead, my patient load doubled.

In a rush of fluid and momentum, a healthy, eight-pound baby girl joined us in the rescue. For a second that seemed like an eternity everything stopped, except for the speeding rescue, as the baby lie still on the stretcher. As I reached for her, a small cry. Then she took her first breath, then another. Then, as I picked her up and dried her, another, louder cry as her skin turned pink.

Adam clamped the umbilical cord, then separated mother and child, but only for an instant.

I handed the package over.

"It's a girl."

If I thought her look from before was priceless, I hadn't seen nothin' yet.

New Me

At the beginning of my shift I often give myself a little inspirational speech.

"I will take this job more seriously."

"I will listen to my patients' complaints."

"I will stop eating everything in sight."

"I will try to learn something new."

"I will not drink a gallon of coffee."

"I will be more professional."

The list changes from shift to shift, but I always start the week with best intentions. Sometimes my resolve lasts for hours. Sometimes minutes. Sometimes I don't even get out the door with my new attitude.

1830 hrs. Dispatched to a women's shelter for a report of back pain. Arrived to find two women, one the patient, the other the patient "advocate." The patient speaks no English and my *Sesame Street* Spanish is not enough to convey the emergency information to the ER.

New Me: "What is the problem?"

Patient (through Advocate): "I have severe back pain."

New Me: "How long have you had this severe back pain?"

Patient: "Many years."

New Me: "And how did this severe back pain begin?"

Patient: "My breasts are too large, I need a breast reduction."

Less New Me: "Your breasts are too large?"

Patient: "The weight of my breasts causes severe back pain."

Even Less New Me: "And how is this even remotely an emergency?"

Patient: "I have back pain."

Old Me: "Get in the truck."

On the official "State of Rhode Island and Providence Plantations Emergency Medical Services" form there is a spot for "Past Medical Conditions." The New Me would have written "Back Pain" on the form. The Old Me is waiting for the phone call from the EMS chief to explain why "Large Breasts" occupies the space relegated for "Past Medical Conditions."

The Solution

I'm running out of men twice as old as me, so the ninety-eight-year-old gentleman who occupied my stretcher was quite a novelty. He wasn't at all what I expected when dispatched to his assisted living facility at 0300 hrs. The call was for chest pain. I wrongly assumed I would be the one feeling most of the pain as I dragged my tired forty-seven-year-old body off the bunk and trudged down the stairs toward the truck. We didn't say much on the way; it's all business in the middle of the night, especially with both of us working overtime with thirty more hours to look forward to.

Our patient lives in a luxury facility, bordering the Providence River. I remember when they built the place; we were amazed at the cost, something like half a million to buy a unit, then another five grand a month to stay there. I always look at the nameplates on the closed doors as we wheel the stretcher down the corridor toward the patient's room. For some reason they always put them in the last room, all the way at the end of the corridor.

"We've got an emergency here, bring him to the last room. And make it snappy!"

Anyway, the names on the plates are indicative of the residents. Dr. and Mrs. Soandso. Admiral Whosit. The Honorable and Mrs. Youknowwho. It's a who's who of the upper crust of Rhode Island society.

Every now and then we pull a cranky old coot out of places like these, but for the most part the fabulously wealthy old folks who need us are polite, gracious, and humble. I'm not sure if life's lessons taught them to be so, or if their demeanor had a lot to do with their success in life.

In the rescue, once all the procedures were done and we rode toward the hospital, Mr. Cohen asked me what I thought about President Obama's pick for the Supreme Court. I thought for a minute and gave him my honest reply.

He grinned mischievously and agreed that the country is "in big trouble." He went on to explain how he grew up in South Providence, right off of Prairie Avenue, and how only Jews and Irish lived there then. Then he explained the division between the German and Austrian Jews and the new Jews, working class folks from Russia and Poland. I mentioned the Irish probably fit in better with the Russians and Poles.

"Half the Jewish people moved to Blackstone Boulevard, the other half stayed," he said.

"The Irish never got the memo," I replied. We just kept on working.

"Strange world," I mentioned, thankful for his historical perspective. "Everybody thinks racism is over now that Obama is in the White House, but I see some strange things. Black folks who have lived here for generations are resentful of the new African immigrants, Dominicans don't like Puerto Ricans, Chinese don't like Koreans, it's a miracle we get anything done."

"I guess things haven't changed since I was a kid," he said. "I wonder if we'll ever figure it out."

"Me too."

I didn't want to leave on a sour note, so as we backed into the ambulance bay at the hospital I told him about the lady who called 911 because her breasts were too large.

Never seen an old guy grin so wide. I guess you never get too old to think about certain things.

At three thirty in the morning the thought of large breasts solving the world's problems seemed almost conceivable.

You Don't Say

Say you are called to a private home for a person who was involved in a previous motor vehicle collision, and say that when you arrive at the address you find a man who you took to the hospital last week for severe complications from renal failure and diabetes, and say that you like this guy, whose luck and health are far worse than your own, and say that this man was in a private ambulance forty-five minutes ago, returning from a dialysis appointment, and say that the private ambulance was involved in a minor collision with a parked vehicle, and say that the ambulance crew neglected to report the incident, even though the patient stated he had been injured.

Just saying.

The Difference

"Attention Engine 3 and Rescue 1, respond to 647 Broad Street for an MVA involving an unresponsive ten-year-old."

That will get you going.

We flew out of the station toward the incident. Engine 3 arrived on scene first and radioed their findings.

"Engine 3 to fire alarm, advise Rescue 1 we have a minor MVA, the ten-year-old's mother wants to 'have her checked.' Alert and conscious, proceed code C."

Code C lets us know the "emergency" is not really an emergency, just somebody's idea of an emergency that really isn't.

An old car had a minor scrape on its side. A middle-aged woman sat in the driver's seat, her daughter occupying the seat behind her.

"You guys are all set," I said to the officer of Engine 3. They went back in service, I stayed with the police and talked to the mom.

"What happened?"

"A guy in a white car sideswiped me and kept on going. I called 911 from my cell phone and asked for the police. I was worried about Monique, she was sleeping in the back seat when the crash happened and didn't wake up."

I looked at Monique. Ten years old, dressed in clean hand-me-downs, a little overweight and the weight of the world on her shoulders from the expression on her face.

"Are you okay?" I asked her. She shook her head, yes. She looked fine, minimal damage to the car, minimal damage to the occupants.

"We could take her to the hospital and have them do an exam if you like," I said to the mom. Monique looked at me as if I had just turned into Frankenstein's monster. I checked my neck to see if any plugs had sprouted. Nope.

"Or, we could do some vital signs and you guys could go home."

Monique liked that idea, so did Mom. Adam went to get the equipment; I sat in the back seat next to the little girl and asked a few questions. Did she know where she was? She did. Did she know what day it was? She did. Did she know who the president was? Boy, did she ever. A smile that could have lit up a coal mine turned her face from plain to beautiful.

As Adam assessed her vital signs, I told her mom, loud enough so the girl could hear, that her daughter was absolutely adorable, and would surely break a lot of hearts as she got older. Monique's smile somehow grew.

We left them, mom and daughter feeling better about themselves than they did before the accident. At least I like to think so.

Please allow me some self-indulgence for a minute, but these are the kind of things that let me to do this job over and over, year after year. I honestly believe that in some small way, by showing a lonely, possibly insecure ten-year-old girl that she had her own brand of beauty that glowed when she smiled, my actions have the chance of making a difference in her life. Maybe I overthink things, perhaps I give myself too much credit, but I envision this girl years from now, looking in her mirror, maybe a little down, but remembering the fireman that said she was adorable and would break some hearts, and just maybe that little positive flow of energy will be enough to keep her from making poor choices that come with low self-esteem and poor body image. Maybe.

It's people like this who help me more than I help them. I need to think I actually do make a difference.

Last Rights?
By the time we got to him he was as good as dead. He had "quit his dialysis months ago," a neighbor informed us, "just gave up."

He was naked, lying on the floor of his one bedroom high-rise apartment. No furniture, a mattress on the floor, no sheets. No food in the fridge. No medications anywhere. No mail. No nothing.

We found his birth certificate. Seventy-nine years old with nothing to show for it. Untreated bedsores covered his back, the skin on his back resembling an alligator's, it was so dry. Urine covered the floor next to him, feces as well.

The faint pulse he had when we entered his world died after a few seconds. The neighbor who called us to check the guy's well-being backed out of the place, the smell a bit too much for somebody not used to such things.

I looked into his dying eyes, saw the light go out, and silently said goodbye.

We performed CPR on the dead body, attempted IVs and intubation, and transported the corpse to the ER, where they continued the lifesaving efforts.

Rest in peace, Lonely Old Man. I'm sorry I had to ruin your last moments.

Pickets
I'm not a fan of picket lines. I don't like walking around in circles, chanting, kind of makes me feel like a chimpanzee.

I don't want to do anything that tarnishes the city of Providence. I want this place to reflect the people I work with, their dedication, honesty, and work ethic. That would be the image I would wish to see written in newspapers, talked about on talk radio, and displayed on television. Instead, the ugly picket line will be headlining things for a while, as the yearly Conference of Mayors visits Providence.

This should be a great moment for the city. National exposure, dignitaries, red carpets and all that. Instead, Providence firefighters and police officers must take to the picket line to bring to attention their situation as it pertains to contract negotiations with the mayor's administration. Make no mistake, picket lines are ugly. There is not one person I know who looks forward to walking the line. When faced with a mayor who is a diabolical, bald-faced liar we have no choice.

The mayor asserts the firefighters refuse to share their healthcare costs. He states, in public and on the air, that firefighters receive unsustainable 6 percent cost of living pension benefits. He claims firefighters are making upwards of $100,000 a year in neighborhoods where families struggle, working three jobs just to make ends meet. He states a lot of things that have no fraction of truth. What makes it worse, he is well aware that he is lying, and thinks he can get away with it. It is an insult to the people of Providence, some working three jobs, and dangerous to attempt to turn the citizens against public safety workers in an effort to bolster his own credibility.

The mayor is losing the battle of public perception, not because the firefighters have a better strategy. He is losing because the firefighters are honest, and right.

If you see a chimpanzee holding a picket sign while watching the news this week don't worry, it's only me. As much as I dislike pickets, I dislike liars even more.

Circle the Wagons

Some idiot got sprayed with mace. I have no idea how or why, all I know is I'm coughing, my face is on fire, and my hands are itchy. Sure, I could have walked away, told him the pain subsides after a while, but a guy was in distress and I helped him. Simple as that. The fact that I got the stuff all over me while cleaning him up is irrelevant. The pain and itching will subside after a while.

A young girl got punched in the face a few nights ago. She stood outside of her three-decker, bleeding from her bottom lip. She offered me money because she didn't have insurance. She told me she was a "dancer" at Cheaters, a notorious adult entertainment club down the road from my station. She opened her purse, a stack of twenties and a bunch of condoms lay inside. The girl was high, confused, and needed help. I helped her. We put her in our truck, dressed her wound, and had her put her money and condoms away. Her ID said she was twenty and lived in Connecticut. Her face said she was sixteen and lived on the streets. Her face was right, her ID a lie.

She was a runaway.

I'd like to think our actions helped her find her way home, whatever hell that might be. I don't know. I do know that I have a job to do, a damned important one. Some day I'm going to get old, and when I look back on my life the proudest moments I'll recall will include those spent as a Providence firefighter.

Right now, as I write this I'm listening to talk radio. Big mistake. My union has decided to picket some big deal mayors' conference in Providence. From the sound of the callers, and the letter writers and people on the street, you would think we invited Satan into our midst to corrupt the youth of the world and pick the pockets of the taxpayers of Providence.

This event will pass, we will picket, life will go on. I'll still be a member of the Providence Fire Department, still stand proud, and still help people when they need it.

It is my honor and privilege to be part of the fire service, most recently serving as a rescue lieutenant. Sometimes we have to circle the wagons and stand together, knowing that ours is a profession unlike no other, whether it is appreciated or not.

Lessons
So, it is time for Grasshopper to try to snatch the pebble from my hand.

The "new guy" has been driving for three months now. In three more months the department will put him in charge of a Providence rescue. Will he be ready? We shall see.

First test: 0715, fifteen minutes into our first shift, cardiac arrest, fifty-five-year-old male.

I failed this test, couldn't relinquish command. Just couldn't. It's one thing to train somebody, another thing altogether to put him into an impossible situation and possibly do more harm to his confidence than good. Our patient was deceased. His extremities were cold to the touch. My guess was he had been gone for at least an hour.

The man's son, who happened to also be a certified nursing assistant, felt his wrist, stated he had a pulse, and then looked to us. The man's wife appeared from a rear bedroom and became hysterical. Many moons ago I may have declared the man dead. Time teaches. The family needed to know everything had been done for their husband, father, son.

I had Adam get the ET tube while we did CPR and monitored the heart. Asystolic. My IV attempts were dismal failures; we arrived at the ER before administering any meds through the tube. The hospital is a teaching hospital, they took over care. He was pronounced dead fifteen minutes later.

The day progressed, I drove for the first time in a while, and my partner handled the patients. He was doing fine until 1430 hrs. when we were called to a Family Services Center for a suicidal fifteen-year-old. Ashley sat in the office with her grandmother, sullen, petulant, and annoyed, everything I was when I was fifteen. She had numerous attempts in her history and suggested to a councilor today that she wanted to die.

Adam sat in the captain's seat while I took the young lady's vital signs. I learned something on this run; I am truly incapable of keeping my big trap shut and letting other people shine.

"You know, Ashley," I said, "I hated being thirteen, fourteen, fifteen, sixteen, seventeen . . . actually I was miserable until I turned forty, only then did I manage to find happiness."

She looked me in the eye, unimpressed.

"Twenty-five is actually pretty good," chimed in my student. "He's just so old he can't remember."

Well, the suddenly animated Ashley and my "student" had a nice little chuckle for themselves as I slinked to the driver's seat and left them in the back.

I looked in my hand as we left the scene.

The pebble was gone.

Welcome to Providence
A lifetime ago a twenty-nine-year-old man stood at attention with sixty-three other trainees listening to the Chief of the Division of Training welcome us to the Providence Fire Department. One by one six training officers introduced themselves to the class. I stood next to the open overhead door on the apparatus floor, a warm summer breeze ruffling

our freshly pressed blue T-shirts and khaki pants as one of the training officers, Lieutenant Thomas, addressed the class, telling us to forget anything we knew, or thought we knew about firefighting. We were there to learn how to do things the Providence Fire Department way, period.

I had been told by people who had been through the rigorous six-month academy to keep my mouth shut, do what I was told, and learn as much as possible. "Whatever you do, don't bring attention to yourself" was the most important thing I could do, I was warned.

As Lieutenant Thomas continued his lecture my eyes wandered to the other side of Reservoir Avenue. There, on the sidewalk, a thirty-year-old woman stood on the side of the road repeatedly lifting her shirt and waving to passing motorists. Without turning my head I watched the spectacle unfold through eyeballs straining to the right, nearly reaching their breaking point. I was sure this was some prank. What else could it be? Eventually the shirt came off. When she sat on the sidewalk and started to take off the rest of her clothes I reluctantly raised my hand, trying to think of how my first words as a Providence firefighter would be remembered.

Lieutenant Thomas looked at me, amazed that one of the trainees had the temerity to raise his hand five minutes into his new career.

"Sir," I said when he glared at me and gave a tiny nod of his head. "I believe a woman across the street needs help."

The lieutenant stood there for a moment, obviously not impressed with my assessment of something he was sure he had seen already, and casually strolled to the open door. The lady's pants were now down around her knees and she was enjoying herself on the sidewalk.

Lieutenant Thomas keyed his mic and asked for police and a rescue to respond to the address for a "woman in distress."

He sauntered back to the front of the class, completely forgetting his opening remarks, shook his head, and finished his speech.

"Welcome to Providence."

For nearly twenty-five years I lived the life of a Providence firefighter. It was a heck of a ride . . .

DOA

"You don't need all that, just bring a sheet."

The captain filled the doorway for a moment, then disappeared.

"Bring it," I said. Adam grabbed the monitor and O2, I carried the "blue bag."

Inside, a man lay dead on his couch. His body was filthy in life; in death it was blue and filthy. A dog whimpered from behind a closed door, week-old food sat on a filthy stove, rotting in a filthy pan in a filthy kitchen. Bugs feasted.

I stood in the doorway that led outside, getting an occasional breath of fresh air, consoling a sobbing woman. I didn't ask if she was related, her grief was proof enough for me that she belonged here. A group of five others hovered around the dead man, the usual chatter, the usual questions, the usual tears.

"Let's go, move it outside," bellowed the captain. "Nothin' here but a dead body and a lot of stink."

Adam told me later I had murder in my eyes.

For some inexplicable reason the people listened to the captain and started to leave.

"Get out of the way," he said to me. "I'm clearing this place out."

He's the fire captain. I'm the rescue lieutenant. We had been dispatched for an unresponsive male. I was in no mood for a pissing contest. I put the sheet over the deceased.

"You don't have to go anywhere," I said to the people as they left the dreadful place.

I can't wait for this shift to end.

Three in, Three Out

So anyway, Providence is home to 180,000 official people. The real number is well over 200,000. Add to that, the 50,000 or so people who fill the city every workday, then come back to party.

Providence runs with six ALS (advanced life support) vehicles and zero BLS (basic life support) vehicles. Six trucks handle 30,000 ALS calls per year and the number is growing. Can't seem to squeeze any more rescues out of the city without taking understaffed firefighters away from the trucks.

What to do?

Nothing. Run, boys, run.

And call for mutual aid.

1430 hrs., a minor fender bender on the south side. Three guys scurry around moving plastering equipment from the trunk of a barely damaged vehicle into the back of a pickup. They see the rescue and stop, holding their backs.

I took two. Rescue 2 took another. A third rescue was called a minute later so the driver of the other car could get on the bandwagon.

Three rescues tied up for no reason other than to fill the pockets of some lawyers and their prey.

Half of Providence's fleet gone in a blink.

Vacation begins in two hours.

Back to Class

It is an awful place, the end of the road. At 0130 we entered through the front door, past the regulars, empty vodka bottles and spent cigarette butts leading the way. Some slept on benches, covered with little more than rags. Others stayed awake, staring into space. We wheeled the stretcher past them on the way to the sixth floor. We had been called to remove an intoxicated man passed out in the corridor.

The elevator seemed smaller than it actually was, stained stainless steel walls, sticky floor, filthy buttons. I tried to hold my breath till floor six but had to exhale around the fourth and breathe in the fetid air before the doors opened into the stench of the sixth floor.

A man lie unconscious on the floor further down the door-lined corridor. Inside the tiny one-room apartments sounds emanated, AC/DC from a portable radio, a man on the phone telling somebody about the unfit living conditions, somebody snoring, somebody vomiting.

I approached the patient, leaned over, and shook him. Cockroaches scurried when he moved, there must have been fifty of them under his body doing God knows what.

"Hey, buddy, wake up," I said, shaking him again. The security guard who escorted us up shook his head and walked away.

"Come on," I said, "we'll help you up."

He opened his eyes and looked at me, did a quick assessment, then tried to stand. He was unsuccessful. We helped him kneel, then rolled him onto the stretcher, covered him with a sheet, and wheeled him down the corridor, into the elevator, to the lobby, and into the night.

On the way to the hospital, as I gathered the necessary information, something hit me in the back of the head like a 2 × 4 swung by a giant.

He was battling cancer, taking chemo and sick as a dog.

He was my age, had a family once.

He was my friend, a long time ago. We went to school together in the seventies. He didn't recognize me. I didn't say anything as I wrote his name on the report. Once, we had similar dreams, similar hopes, and similar ambitions.

His fell apart. Mine came true.

I've done seventeen runs in seventeen hours. An hour ago I thought I had it tough.

Loss

My friend Bill, a captain on the Providence Fire Department, lost his son early this morning. When we were neighbors I'd see them often, getting ready to take the kids camping, playing catch, making a skateboard ramp, just a great family man doing all the right things.

If you have children, take them aside, hug them whether they want it or not, look them in the eye and tell them you love them. Then let them go and hope they stay safe. And do it often.

I spent much of last night walking with my oldest, Danielle. We walked her dog to the beach near our home, came back and rescued a squirrel that was trapped in a downspout. It's a goofy little memory that seems so much more important now.

My wife is refinishing a chest of drawers for "the baby" (she's twenty-eight). It's a long process, painting each drawer, sanding, putting a faux finish on it, sending a picture for approval, then proceeding to the next step. It will be beautiful when finished.

We have each other. We are still creating memories. Every day is precious.

Nobody knew that more than Bill and his wife. They created enough memories to carry them through this tragedy.

Poverty

On a busy street, with the front door four feet from the street, lives a family of five. They rent one of the apartments. It's small. Two bedrooms, a kitchen without a table, and a small living room. A bathroom small enough to serve as a closet in a different place is filled with tools to help a handicapped child.

His father carries him out. He's five. His teeth are separated by quarter-inch spaces but clean. They protrude from his white lips, almost like a set of joke teeth you would buy at a novelty store. Only this is no joke. The boy's skin is grey. He hasn't eaten in two days and has been vomiting nonstop. The father lays the boy on the stretcher. I can only watch him, stunned. I've never seen a living child look so dead. He is breathing. He looks at me when I come close, looks me in the eye and smiles. I put the blood pressure cuff around his tiny arm and it begins to inflate. The child doesn't flinch.

His mother enters the back of the rescue holding her daughter. She is one year old, beautiful dark curls surround her healthy, chubby face. She cries, nonstop. She too has been sick for days. What little Spanish I know is enough. These kids are sick. The boy has cerebral palsy. The girl is healthy. Another child stays at home with his father as I take the mom and two kids to the hospital.

She is a pretty woman, probably no more than twenty. Her hair is tied back with an elastic band. Her clothes are clean, a long skirt and peasant blouse, brightly colored. The sandals she wears look good on her, but are at least five years out of fashion. She doesn't mind, at least she has shoes on her feet. Her toenails are carefully painted to match her clothes. A small luxury in an otherwise difficult life.

She smiles at her son as we ride together toward the hospital. He is in tough shape but smiles back. If anybody needed medical care, it is him.

She gives me two cards. I callously refer to them as "the Key to the Kingdom," sometimes. The cards represent free healthcare for the poor. A lot of people abuse the system, our Medicare budget takes up a third of the state of Rhode Island's revenue.

I copy the information on the state report, occasionally looking at the kids.

I can't help but be proud of my standing as an American citizen, able and willing to help those so desperately in need. If the tables were turned, and I was born in Mexico and impoverished, I hope I would have the courage to brave it all and make the journey to where a better life existed for my family, immigration laws be damned.

Relentless
The calls keep coming. Every time I put the truck in service we get sent to another call. Now and then an hour or so passes without a run, mostly it's just one after the other. They are starting to blend into one. Nine years ago, when I decided to transfer from Engine 9 to Rescue 1, I made a promise: when I stopped seeing my patients as people it would be time to get off the rescue.

I haven't seen a lot of people lately. Just calls. And they keep coming.

Filter
He sat on the stretcher; skinny kid, good thing too or the bullet that grazed him would have been in his body. I let him talk on his cell phone en route to the ER, didn't bother me much, it sounded like he was talking to his mom, who was pretty upset. He repeated over and over he was okay, was just standing there talking with his friend when some guys came upon them and opened fire. He was concerned about his friend, nobody knew where he was.

We got him to the hospital and were preparing to leave when another call came in to the same location for another gunshot victim.

Shit.

We sped out of the ER fully expecting the worst.

"Rescue 1, expedite," came over the radio.

We were on scene a minute later.

Lying facedown in the dirt, head up against a chain-link fence, next to a swimming pool was our first patient's friend. I rolled him over, felt for pulses, looked into his dead eyes, noticed the holes in his torso, and realized we were too late.

I focused on the sound of the pool filter, the water soothing as screams, sobs, and shouting filled the air around us.

Eternity

"Rescue 1, respond to 7265 Progress Lane, at the Adult Video News for a man down."

I fumbled for my radio, sitting in the charger next to my bunk. The indicator light was still red, must not have been out for long. I stood, felt the pains run up my legs, felt the familiar stiffness in my back and neck, and did a quick stretch. I took a deep breath. Dragon fire. Should I brush? How would the "man down" feel about his rescuer doing a little bird bath and breath refreshment before rushing to his aid?

I popped a piece of Trident in, because it freshens your breath while whitening your teeth, rubbed the bed head out of my scalp, and hit the pole. Three minutes later, we stopped the truck in front of the X-rated novelty store. A woman ran out, shocked.

"He's in there!" she said, pointing into the dark doorway. The sun had barely risen. Some days, dawn is beautiful and refreshing, others, just downright creepy.

"He's not supposed to be in there!" she continued, hiding behind me as I walked into the empty building. I keyed the mic.

"Rescue 1 to fire alarm, have the police respond here, possible trespasser."

"Where is he?"

"In the back."

"What's he doing?"

"Just laying there."

I approached the back of the store where the private viewing booths were.

"Which one?"

She pointed to a closed door. I wanted to walk out and forget the whole thing. Instead, I opened the door.

A man lay on the floor, dead. His face was plastered to the stained carpeting. The last video he ever saw was over. I reached in, felt for a pulse that I knew wouldn't be there. Ice cold.

"Rescue 1 to fire alarm, time on scene and a police sergeant."

"0622 hrs., Rescue 1. Police have been notified."

When the cops got there I told them time of death 0622. In reality, he died around 2300 hrs., alone, watching porn in a dirty booth on a skeevy block surrounded by deviants. He looked to be around fifty. Fifty years of life, family, kids, maybe church, might have been a coach, a teacher, a firefighter, a priest . . . who knows.

All I know is his last act is probably not how he wanted to be remembered for all eternity.

A Little Fire

0415 hrs. *"Attention Engines 2, 7, 12, Ladders 7 and 4, Special Hazards, Rescue 3, and Battalion 3 a stillbox."* A "stillbox" refers to a call made by a human, rather than a mechanized box alarm. Bright light floods the fire stations at Branch Avenue, North Main Street, and Admiral Street. Firefighters immediately rise from their bunks and slide the brass poles.

Within twenty seconds they are dressed in their turnout gear and mounting their apparatus.

The PA system blares: *"Attention Engines 2, 7, 12, Ladders 7 and 4, Special Hazards, Rescue 3, and Battalion 3, respond to 63 Douglas Avenue for a reported building fire, possibly occupied."*

Immediately, fire trucks are on their way. Hundreds of hours spent studying streets ensure there will be no mistake; the trucks will arrive in the shortest time possible. The first-in companies consist of four firefighters from Engine 2 and three on Ladder 7.

0420 hrs. *"Engine 2 on scene, three-story wood frame, fire on the second floor, occupied. Code red."*

Code red signals that a working fire has been found at the location. Air packs are donned, tools readied, and nerves steadied. Sirens echo in the empty streets.

A fire rages on the second floor of a tenement house. The first-floor tenant who discovered the fire and made the first 911 call relays information that people, a single man on the second and an elderly couple on the third, are still in the house.

The driver of Engine 2 stops his vehicle fifty feet past the fire building, transfers power from the transmission to the pump, gets out of the cab, and prepares to feed the attack companies the water necessary to extinguish the blaze. He opens the tank-to-pump valve, throttles up, and gets ready for commands. Engine 2's officer, the incident commander for now, is sizing up the fire ground, planning the attack until the chief arrives and establishes Douglas Command. Strict rules will be followed: the incident command system, a nationally used method of organizing emergency responses of all sizes, must be used. The remaining two firefighters from Engine 2 stretch 250 feet of 1¾-inch attack line toward the rear door, knowing that it will lead to the second-story stairs.

"Battalion 3 on scene, establishing Douglas Command."

"Ladder 7 on scene."

"Rescue 3 on scene, establishing EMS sector."

The rescue is ready to triage victims and call for additional help if needed. The ladder company is prepared to "get the roof."

The driver of the ladder truck slows down two hundred feet from the fire. Utility wires, parked cars, and trees obstruct his path toward the roof. The officer leaves the cab and finds a good spot to set up. There is no second chance. A wrong placement of the ladder will severely hamper the firefighting efforts. He directs the driver toward the front of the house, stopping him at the perfect location.

The driver switches the truck from drive to PTO, which enables the aerial ladder to begin operations. He and the third firefighter get ready to raise the ladder to the roof. Outriggers must be lowered and secured, the ladder unlocked, then raised. One person handles the controls, the other watches the progress.

The officer is at the rear of the house helping to force the door open. Once the ladder is in place, rising fifty-five feet between utility wires and through tree branches, the firefighters load up their tools, a quick-vent saw, axes and poles, and begin to climb. Inside the house heat and gasses are accumulating, filling the space. Ventilation is imperative. Failure is not an option.

0423 hrs. *"Engine 7 on scene, establishing water supply."*

The second due engine is responsible for water supply. Its crew finds the closest hydrant, five hundred feet away, and stops the truck. The officer and one of the firefighters get out, take two lengths of three-inch hose from the hose bed and the hydrant dressing gear, and signal the driver to go. Engine 7 rolls toward Engine 2, trailing the supply lines without which no fire will be extinguished.

0425 hrs. *"Engine 2 to pump operator, charge my line!"*

The firefighter at the pump expertly pulls levers and gates, and then watches as the initial 250-foot attack line fills with water and slithers toward the rear door, up the stairs into the toxic atmosphere, and toward the pipe. Engine 2 carries five hundred gallons of water, enough for about three minutes. The officer of Ladder 7 has located the sleeping occupant of the second floor and is helping him out of the house. The firefighters from Engine 2 man the line and hit the fire, plunging the apartment into darkness. The heat and smoke are unbearable, even to firefighters fully dressed in gear.

The fire is stubborn, more water needed.

0426 hrs. *"Special Hazards on scene."*

"Battalion 3 to Special Hazards, start a primary search of the second floor."

"Ladder 4 on scene."

"Battalion 3 to Ladder 4, primary on the third."

The Hazards and Ladder 4 turn in their packs and enter the building. The man from the second floor is safe and in the rescue vehicle. Another rescue is called for transport.

The battle rages. On the steeply pitched roof, the two firefighters from Ladder 7 straddle the peak, start the quick-vent saw that starts on the first pull—no accident; every piece of equipment is thoroughly checked daily—and begin ventilating. A proper hole needs to be four feet by four feet. The two firefighters from Engine 7 have "dressed the hydrant," removed all three ports, attached a hydrant gate to the large-diameter opening, an extra port to one of the smaller ports and a three-inch feeder line to the other. One waits by the hydrant, the officer starts toward Engine 2. Connections to the water supply must be made. Firefighters and possibly civilians are committed inside the burning structure. If the water supply is interrupted a successful outcome will be in doubt.

"Engine 12 on scene."

Four firefighters from Engine 12 arrive. They immediately stretch another attack line from the rear of Engine 2 and start toward the rear door to back up Engine 2.

"Engine 2 to Engine 7, turn in the hydrant."

The firefighter manning the hydrant receives the message and turns the spindle fourteen revolutions, fully opening the valve. The feeders fill and make way toward the pump, which is beginning to cavitate, every drop from the tank gone. Just in time water supply is established. The fight goes on.

With the water supply established, the crew of Engine 7 now takes another attack line from Engine 2 and enters the door toward the third floor. They fight their way up and join the crew of Ladder 4, who have just finished their primary search of the third-floor apartment. Thankfully, this time there was nobody home.

The fire has spread through the walls and is now in the loft. Inside, the fire crews feel something shift and know the roof is open. The heat and smoke clear just enough to make the fight bearable. Walls and ceilings are opened by pulling the plaster with poles. Fire is found and quickly extinguished. Two members from Special Hazards are now in the basement cutting the electric supply, the other two are assisting with vertical ventilation, opening windows and doors. Once the electric supply is off, ground ladders must be raised to the second- and third-floor windows to supply a secondary means of egress.

0500 hrs. Now the dangerous part begins. The flames are knocked down, but sparks and embers hide everywhere — inside walls, in every nook and cranny imaginable. Every remnant of fire must be extinguished or there will be a rekindle.

0556 hrs. Sunrise. The exhausted firefighters converge around Engines 7 and 2, repacking the hundreds of feet of hose. It was a good job: nobody was injured, the house damaged but saved.

0600 hrs. A man walks his dog past the firefighters.

"What happened?" he asks.

"Fire on the second floor," somebody responds.

The man stands there, looks at the house, takes in the minor damage visible from the outside, and asks smugly, "All this to put out a little fire." He shakes his head in disdain and walks away.

Night Terrors

She had entered a place she may not have wanted to go. Sixteen years old, visiting a local college with a friend, when a light went on in her mind. The things we keep there, stored in a safe place, are a mystery. It may be better that way.

Part of the college's program included a guest hypnotist. One hundred and fifty high school juniors and seniors were in attendance. One hundred and forty-nine enjoyed the mass hypnosis, got a few chills, had a few laughs, and went on to the next phase of the orientation. Ellie didn't come back. She stayed in a trance.

Rescue 1 was dispatched to the campus for an emotional female. Our patient, a pretty student dressed in a summer dress and sandals, sat on a couch in the security office next to the hypnotist, who coolly tried to talk her back from the place he put her. He made way when we arrived. I knelt in front of Ellie, thinking she was having us on and getting a huge kick out of all the attention, and introduced myself. She stared blankly ahead, sobbing uncontrollably, hyperventilating. Her breathing rate had increased to sixty breaths a minute, she was close to passing out.

The hypnotist seemed genuinely concerned, but just as genuinely relieved that somebody else was now responsible. I thought it prudent to clear the room out; it was stifling and oppressive.

"Do you know where you are?" I asked, looking deep into her eyes. Nothing. She just cried and continued hyperventilating. I took one of her hands into mine. She flinched and tried to pull back. I held on.

"I'm not going to hurt you, I want you back," I said. She relaxed, stared into my eyes, and kept crying. Then, the intensity of her sorrow and terror increased, her body was racked with shudders; she was truly terrified.

"Ellie," I said as quietly as I could, "how old are you?"

She looked at me for a long time, her hand moist with sweat. She honestly couldn't remember. I remembered a technique I learned a while ago, Emotional Freedom Technique. It is similar to acupressure, tapping on different points of the body that are connected to certain meridians and central nervous system trigger points. I didn't think it would hurt so I started gently tapping the inside of her hand while talking to her.

"You're breathing too fast, Ellie. You have to slow down. Talk with me when you breathe. One, two, one, two." I said "one" upon inhaling, "two" when exhaling, and continued tapping her hand. It was fast but I was persistent. The group counselor stood nearby, thinking I was mad, and my partner for the night, Mark, tapped his foot impatiently, but I thought I was on to something. Ellie's breathing started to slow down after a few minutes, but she was still far gone.

"One, two, one, two." Slower and slower until she was down to twelve breaths a minute. I tried to pull my hand away, this time it was she who wouldn't let go.

Unfortunately, that was as close as I could get. I tried for another five minutes to get her to come to. She still couldn't answer any of our questions, but at least she was breathing normally. It was a small victory, but not the result I wanted. I had hoped she could rejoin her friends and have some fun while visiting the school. She should have been with the rest of the kids, clowning around, making connections, and living the best years of her life instead of lying on a stretcher on her way to the hospital for a psychological evaluation.

The counselor came with us and contacted Ellie's mom. I took the phone and asked a few questions. Was Ellie on any medications? No. Did she have psychological problems? No. Has anything like this ever happened before?

Ellie was completely gone now. Her mother heard her daughter crying in the background and said it was like going back in time to twelve years ago when her daughter suffered with "night terrors" for a while.

"She sounds like she is five again," said her mom as goose bumps crawled up my arms. Ellie still looked directly at me, into me, and continued to cry, body-wrenching, heart-stopping sorrow. I hung up the phone after asking her mom to take it easy, her daughter was in good hands and would be safe until she got there. She came from White Plains, New York, about five hours away, and was on her way while I had her on the phone.

We arrived at the children's hospital and told the story to the skeptical triage nurse. It wasn't long before she too was mystified by the patient, who was now pulling her tongue, trying to tear it from her mouth.

All this from a kid who never exhibited any abnormalities, left New York that morning as happy as can be, and ended up in a hospital after hypnotist's trick went badly.

I checked on her the next day. She was gone, released to her family. They did a thorough neurological workup and found nothing amiss.

I don't think she will ever return to Providence, and I'm positive she will never get hypnotized again.

Good luck, Ellie. I hope the demons stay at bay, or better yet, you find the courage to confront them, and send them away for good.

Fools

She sat on the front steps of her home, overnight bag packed, cigarette in hand.

We stopped the truck. She kept on smoking. And sitting.

"Did you call 911?" I asked, nicely enough.

"Yup." Another drag from the cigarette.

"Why did you call?"

"I need to go to the hospital."

I stretched my neck and peered around the corner of her house. Lo and behold, THE HOSPITAL!

"Get in."

Slowly, ever so slowly she finished her cigarette as I stood there. Now, at one time anger would have invaded my sleep-deprived mind and all sorts of unsavory things would have spewed from my bitter lips. No more. The minions of Providence have cured me of my emotionally charged rants. I'm simply a beaten man. I picked up her overnight bag, carried it into the back of the rescue, had a seat, and waited. Eventually, she joined me, now wearing headphones, the music so loud I could hear the song clearly.

We didn't have long, so I got right to the point.

"Why do you need to go to the hospital?"

She graced me by glancing in my direction, lowered the headphones, and said, "WHAT?"

"Why do you need to go to the hospital?" I repeated.

"I need to be seen."

She reached into her bag, pulled out a Lean Cuisine, opened the tinfoil top, picked up a plastic fork, and dug in.

Surely God tested me.

"Why do you need to be seen?"

"I'll tell THEM when we get there." The phones went back on, I was dismissed.

We backed into the ambulance bay. Stephanie, my driver for the night, opened the side door, fuming, ready to rumble. I smiled and shook my head, no. The three of us walked in together, me keeping the two women separated. Later, Steph had me rolling when she told me they almost needed another rescue for some "black on black" crime.

I told the triage nurse exactly what happened, without embellishing, even a little. Our patient had exquisite hearing, apparently, as she shouted from the other side of the ER for me to "stop talking behind my back."

She continued to interrupt.

"I was not uncooperative!"

"Yes, you were."

"YOU were uncooperative."

"No, I wasn't."

"I don't need to tell no ambulance driver nothing'."

"I wasn't driving."

"Just do your job."

"I couldn't, you were uncooperative."

She wanted to continue. I didn't care. The twenty or so patients in the ER looked on, bewildered. I continued giving my report.

"Her appetite isn't compromised, and her ability to smoke intact. Other than that, I have no idea."

"Ain't no use arguing with no fool!" she said, and put her headphones back on.

I couldn't have agreed more.

Birthday Party

Under a highway, next to some railroad tracks they made their camp. It was her birthday; she turned thirty-three today. He bought her a cake and a tube of frosting so she could write her name on top. Nobody had ever bought her a cake he told us as the IV went in. An Amtrak train sped past, fifteen feet from where we worked, whipping up pebbles and dust. The wind it created seemed to draw you closer, but that is probably just an illusion. The fear of death is always close when standing next to a speeding train.

They decided to party, he bought some heroin. It was the least he could do for his girl. Generous by nature, he let her have more, nice guy that he is. Put her right into respiratory failure. He tried on his own to revive her, slapped her, and dragged her into the rain, soaking her, picked her up, crossed the tracks and tried carrying her up the twenty-foot ledge we had just climbed down. He failed there, at the foot of the ledge, and used his cell to call 911. At forty-eight years old, there simply wasn't enough strength left to do the job.

Once the Narcan kicked in she was able to get up and help us as we helped her climb the steep hill toward the rescue. He carried the cake, the red scribble that was supposed to say her name nothing but a smudge, washed away by the mist. I wondered if she had died there, under a bridge, in the rain, twenty feet below the rest of us, if her life would have been as easily obscured. Gone, just another junkie; homeless and abandoned.

She cried then, once she left the make-believe world under the bridge and entered reality. Her pupils remained pinpoint and her breathing rate slow, but I just didn't have the heart to administer more Narcan and take the little high that remained away.

Absolutely

As some of you have noticed, I've grown weary of life on Rescue 1 and the EMS system as we know it. The thought of leaving this behind after eight years has become almost an obsession. An opening on Engine 10 on Broad Street has appeared and will disappear in a few days. I would be working in the same neighborhood on an ALS engine company as a firefighter. I did firefighting for ten years on various trucks in the city and enjoy it. The people who work at Broad Street are the best; I've been working alongside them for years.

So what the hell is keeping me here?

Stubborn Swede?

Yup.

The glory?

Hahahahah!

The loot?

Partly true.

Some EMTs and paramedics will be amazed to learn that in Providence the people assigned to the rescues are better compensated than the people on the fire trucks.

Alas, the real reason I'm staying is simple. I love it. It doesn't happen often, or nearly often enough, but when I am able to make a connection with one of my patients, and truly understand what is ailing them, be it physical or emotional, and help them get better, an indescribable feeling of well-being takes over, something not available in a bottle or a pill, and makes me feel truly alive. The place I feel God's presence the most is in the back of Rescue 1, when despair, chaos, and heartache lose the battle to caring, competence, and healing.

It is at these times I feel truly blessed, and all the nonsense that comes with the territory becomes minuscule in the big picture.

Will the drunks continue to call?

Of course.

Will people consider us their free ride to the hospital?

I'm sure.

Will I still get six calls after midnight?

No doubt.

Will I find satisfaction in spite of everything that is wrong?

Absolutely.

Shutout

The gods are smiling on me and all is well in the universe. For the first time this century (well maybe not the first, but the first I can remember), Rescue 1 pitched a shutout after midnight last night. Four calls between 1800 hrs. and 2359, then lights out. Zilch, zero, nothing!

Just when you think you have had enough, a little tidbit comes your way and lets you think anything is possible. A little dramatic I'm sure, but what the heck, I really needed that!

Beatings, Babies, and Butter

"Did they put butter on your head?"

She looked at me like I was crazy. Thirteen years old, tough little girl, just got jumped by a crowd of people. There was a fight planned, supposedly one on one. Two girls settling whatever differences they had. Not my idea of the right thing to do, but then I don't live in the inner city.

"Butter. Smear it on your head."

Her face was scratched and bruised, shiny. She lay on the backboard looking up, the c-collar uncomfortable but bearable. A few minutes ago she sat on a chair on a porch on Adelaide Avenue, surrounded by family members. There must have been fifteen women crowding her, speaking rapid-fire Spanish. I stood at the bottom of the steps and finally made eye contact. She wanted out of there.

"Why would I smear butter on my head?" she asked.

"Because, last night we picked up a baby who had fallen out of her baby carriage. Her mother smeared a pound of butter on her head before we got there, I think to reduce the swelling. Her hair was all clumped up and sticky, she looked like a little alien had landed."

I did my best alien impersonation. The two ladies on the bench cracked up as they watched their sullen thirteen-year-old laugh like a little girl again. It was nice to see her without the game face these kids have to wear to survive.

And I thought the butter was a waste of time. It may not have worked for the baby last night, but it did wonders for Auriella.

Rock On

I've been waiting. Every time I turn on the radio I listen for one of those roll down the windows, spark up a fatty, step on the gas, drive to the ocean rip off my clothes and dive into a wave rock anthems that make my ears bleed, face melt, heart beat faster and sing out loud, one of those songs that makes me think that for as long as this lasts anything is possible.

Allow me to take a little trip back in time, names and dates are probably confused but what the heck, the party was in full swing:

Summer of '70, "Jumpin' Jack Flash" by the Stones.

Summer of '71, "Saturday Night's Alright for Fighting," Elton John (yeah I know).

Summer of '72, "Ballroom Blitz," the Sweet.

Summer of can't remember, "Won't Get Fooled Again," The Who, "Born to Run," Springsteen, "Train Kept a Rollin'," Aerosmith, "More Than a Feeling," Boston, "Rock On," David Essex, "School's Out," Alice Cooper, "You've Got Another Thing Comin'," Judas Priest, "Freebird," Lynyrd Skynyrd, "Back in Black," AC/DC, "Jailbreak," Thin Lizzy,

"Smells Like Teen Spirit," Nirvana, "Panama," Van Halen, "Alive," Pearl Jam, "Sweet Child o' Mine," Guns N' Roses . . . I could go on but I have to go.

Anybody else remember?

These songs transcended age, culture, and taste. They were everywhere, you couldn't miss them. I miss that stuff, everything seems so compartmentalized now.

One good song brings so many people together. I hope somebody comes up with one soon. We need it.

Skunkin' Dog

I'm at the ER. I just brought a girl in who claims somebody ran her over then pulled a gun on her. The person who allegedly pulled the gun, I just found out, is in the waiting room.

My phone rings.

Saint Misusmorse: "There's skunks in the yard."

Me: "It's three o'clock in the morning."

Saint Misusmorse: "It doesn't matter, there's six skunks prowling around the bird feeder."

Me: "We need a skunkin' dog."

Saint Misusmorse: "What is a skunkin' dog?"

Me: "A dog that kills skunks."

Saint Misusmorse: "And where do you suppose I get a skunkin' dog?"

Me: "Catch a skunk, kill it, tie it to a four-foot length of rope. Bring the dead skunk to the dog pound. Drag it in front of the cages. Whichever dog barks loudest is our skunkin' dog."

Saint Misusmorse: "Bring home some mothballs."

The phone goes dead.

I think this place is making me crazy.

Walk Away

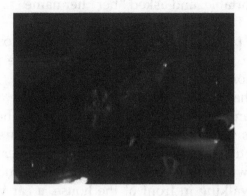

Airbags and seat belts are beautiful things. Scrapes and bruises, some neck and back pain, and a few lacerations beat body bags every time.

New Sheriff in Town

"Rescue 1, Respond to 82 Lincoln Street for a pedestrian struck."

"Rescue 1, on the way."

82 Lincoln Street borders one of the local colleges, plenty of kids walking around and plenty of kids driving like morons to run them over. We hit the lights and siren and started toward the incident. From the top of the street I saw three police cars. We approached the scene expecting the worst.

"Where is everybody?" I asked one of the cops who stood next to his cruiser.

He pointed at one of the houses.

"She's in there."

I entered the house; it is a group home for teens. A young girl sat on a kitchen chair, looking annoyed. Before I said a word a woman handed me some paperwork and informed me I would be taking "her" to the hospital. I ignored the woman, leaned over the chair, close but not close enough to be uncomfortable, and asked "her" her name.

"Ashley," she said. "I'm not even hurt."

"It's our policy that clients be taken to the hospital," said the woman, again attempting to hand me the paperwork. Again I ignored her.

"What happened, Ashley?" I asked. She sat a little straighter and brushed her bangs away from her eyes. Big brown eyes that had seen more in sixteen years than most see in a lifetime. I know why these kids live here and it has little to do with them. Some people just shouldn't have kids.

"I was walking in front of the house, a car was turning around and brushed into me. They're making a big deal out of nothing."

"I'm getting my supervisor, wait here," the woman told me, holding a phone to her ear.

We walked out, Steve, Ashley, and me. I told Ashley not to worry, I just needed to get her complaint and vital signs documented and make sure she truly wasn't hurt. Inside the rescue we all relaxed, took her vitals, and talked a bit. She told us her mother "just lost it" and she shouldn't be living here but had no choice, for now anyway. We finished our assessment and returned to the house. The woman with the phone waited.

"It is our policy that any client that is injured be transported to the hospital to be checked," she said, victoriously.

"Didn't you get the memo?" I asked.

"The memo?"

"Yes, the memo. The one that says the Providence Fire Department does not now, ever did, or ever will worry about yours or anybody else's "policies." If a person is sick or injured or needs emergency medical treatment, we will decide the best course of action. The best course of action here is done. Ashley is not injured. If you feel she needs to be seen by an emergency room doctor to confirm that, I suggest you find a way to get her there."

Ashley loved it.

I've got to admit I kind of liked it too. When I decided to stay on Rescue 1, I also decided that I was going to have to make some changes.

I am a firefighter and an EMT, and a lieutenant with one of the best fire departments in the country. It's about time I remembered that and started acting like one.

Nice Finish
The captain of Engine 14 met me at the bottom of the stairs.

"We're going to need a board."

It was the last call of the day for all of us, at least we hoped so. Shift change happens at 1700 hrs., this call came in at 1645. It was a blistering hot summer afternoon; everybody had been running all day.

I walked up the stairs toward the third floor, the heat increased with every step. It started at 85 degrees, ended around 110. The stairway was cluttered, boxes, bureaus, and things made the tight spot tighter still. Three firefighters waited for me in the third-floor apartment. A thirty-year-old woman was on her back, crying. One leg went straight out, the other curved at an impossible angle at her knee.

"This isn't going to be easy," said Greg, one of the firefighters. Matt knelt next to the patient getting her blood pressure and pulse while Dan attempted to secure the injured leg. The woman screamed every time he touched her.

The captain came back in, carrying a backboard that we have set up for situations such as these, straps in place, blocks secured, ready to go. A split stretcher would have been nice but the powers that be decided we should be without them.

"Are you allergic to any medications?" I asked, praying morphine wasn't on the list. She didn't speak English, luckily her brother was able to translate. No allergies.

"She was putting the baby on the bed when she lost her balance and fell. I don't know how she did it but she managed to keep the baby from getting hurt."

I love moms.

I had to go back down the stairs to get the morphine. We have it double locked and then locked again.

"We'll take care of this," said the captain. I noticed he was wearing gloves, as were his guys.

A few minutes later I came back with the pain meds. I administered 8 mg IM and waited. After a few minutes we were able to move the patient onto the backboard, gently secure her to it, immobilize the knee and leg, and carry her down the three flights of narrow stairs. Once I gave the morphine the firefighters took over, and did a fantastic job getting the patient extricated. It was a potentially horrible situation made better by competent people who ignored the time, focused on the patient, put egos aside, and did their job.

Fire-based EMS works when everybody knows their job and isn't afraid to get dirty doing it. The crew of Engine 14 had a combined total of over eighty years' experience in a busy urban fire department. It is a pleasure working with them.

At five thirty we were ready to roll. The captain asked if we needed help at the ER. His crew was willing to see this through. I thanked them instead, and shut the rear doors. The patient and her brother rode with me in the back. She didn't feel a thing, and thanked me in English once we had her settled in at the hospital.

What's Next
It's Friday morning, 0820 hrs. I've been here since 1700 hrs. last night and won't be free until 0700 hrs. tomorrow morning. Typical Thursday night, three intoxicated men, a seventeen-year-old girl who was released from the hospital two hours prior to calling 911 again because the medication they gave her for pulled muscles weren't working (the family lived half a mile from the ER, followed in the car . . . both times), a building fire, a thirty-nine-year-old female vomiting, and a guy sleeping next to the highway. I'm sure there are a few more but they were as unmemorable as the others.

The cost for all of this emergency medicine is staggering. Some day I'm going to do a running total of the costs incurred by the people who call 911 during a typical shift. Mr. Cynical himself will probably be amazed.

Washington wants to fix the health care system. They should start at the emergency room.

Just for giggles, whatever happens next will be my next post. I'm fairly certain it will be uneventful, but the beauty of this job is the unknown. I may be entering the twilight zone. Or not. We shall see.

Stay tuned!

Abused Angels
1022 hrs., Rescue 1 responds to 622 Elmwood Avenue for an intoxicated male. This is an everyday occurrence. The McCauley House is run by some truly great, patient, benevolent people. Hundreds line up daily outside year-round for the free lunches. A few of their clientele are chronic, homeless alcoholics. They are treated with kindness there, given a warm meal and, more important than that, some respect.

We respond to the address. Two "regulars," a man and woman, both in their early fifties, sit on a wall keeping each other upright. Today, the man is more intoxicated than the woman.

"I'm doing good," she says, giving me a high five as I help her companion to his feet. He is dead weight, about 175 pounds of a body that barely functions. His clothes are clean, he must have gotten new ones from the hospital. Yesterday he was filthy.

"I'll be there in a little while," the woman tells him and gets in line for the free lunch.

Partners

Six months ago, Adam showed up at Rescue 1 to begin his six-month detail. He started on a Sunday night. By week's end we had survived a bloody suicide attempt, a ten-year-old in cardiac arrest who almost made it, and a couple of shootings that didn't. You get to know your partner fast in Providence.

I'll be getting another partner soon; Adam will be greatly missed. Engine 7 is waiting for him; hopefully he'll get tired of that old horse and find his way home. It seems I'm constantly losing friends to the red trucks. Mike went to Engine 15, Renato is at Engine 11, now this. I suppose I'll survive.

He worried about his upcoming wedding, and who to and not to invite. You can't invite everybody, some people you want there just have to be passed over. I remember saying that he shouldn't feel obligated to invite me, that the tradition of inviting your officer to things like this could be waived, considering his newness to the job and all. At the time it seemed like a logical thing to say. Months later I couldn't imagine being left out.

Meg and Adam were married Sunday at Whispering Pines at Alton Jones. They met there some years ago when they worked as camp counselors. The ceremony was held outside at the edge of a pond. Meg was stunning. Somehow she mixed elegance with an outdoorsy sparkle that was absolutely natural, charming, and perfect. I loved that she didn't wear shoes.

I've never seen two people more in sync. They move together, smile at the same time, walk in stride, and are filled with that magic everybody wants.

Thank you, Meg and Adam, for having us share your day. It was a refreshing breath of love, honesty, and joy. I am proud to know you.

Standing Order
Patient #1, a fifty-year-old male, calls from a pay phone outside a bar at one thirty in the morning, states he has chest pain. The rescue arrives, the patient tells the crew to take him to St. Farthest. Apparently, St. Closest, a world-class hospital, doesn't treat our patient right. He refuses to cooperate, won't give any information other than he has been drinking all day and is now having chest pain, severity 10 on a 1-to-10 scale.

Patient #2, an eighty-three-year-old male, sits on the floor in his bathroom at three fifteen in the morning holding the toilet bowl to keep from slumping over. His wife of forty-some years calls 911 for assistance getting him up. The rescue arrives, finds the patient is undergoing chemo to treat lung cancer, is extremely weak and dehydrated. His treatment thus far has been at St. Farthest.

Patient #1 is treated and transported to St. Closest, much to his dismay.

Patient #2 is treated and transported to St. Farthest. No questions asked.

Our protocols clearly state that emergency personnel transport patients without delay to the appropriate hospital emergency facility.

Both patients were treated appropriately.

Rescue 1 has a standing operating procedure: nice guys *never* finish last!

At Peace

The guys from Engine 10 were doing CPR when we arrived. "Asystole," said Kraz.

He lay on the floor next to a hospital bed in the front room of an ordinary house on an ordinary street in Providence. The diaper he wore was clean; the inflated plastic bags that were wrapped around his hands to prevent scratching were new.

"Who found him?" I asked. Three or four family members stood outside the room, afraid.

"He was awake ten minutes ago," said a twenty-year-old woman.

"Is there any paperwork or records?"

"What do you mean?" She was nervous, shaking as she watched the firefighters behind me move her grandfather onto a backboard and continue pumping his chest and breathe for him.

"Did he have any wishes should something like this happen?" The guys had him ready to go.

"No bracelets or necklace," said Bill.

"I know things are a little hectic," I said to the girl, "but I could really use some information. Is there a folder or something from the hospital?"

She handed me a thick folder from the visiting nurse company that visited every day. No advance directive. I scanned the room, looking for anything that would allow me to let this man die in peace. Nothing. A picture on a wall showed my patient in 1967, dressed in a South Vietnamese military uniform, smiling, holding a rifle. His name and date of birth were written below. On a dresser were some medications. I put them in a bag, copied the information from the wall, and left the home.

Inside the rescue we worked the code. An IV was established, epi and atropine administered, CPR continued when a rhythm didn't materialize. We had the defibrillator pads attached. I looked at the flat line on the monitor after each drug was pushed, hoping it stayed flat. It didn't seem fair, he had fought enough.

My intubation attempt was unsuccessful; we rolled toward the ER, CPR all the way. Though I thought the effort doomed from the start, my training took over. We did all we could.

The medical team had assembled prior to our arrival. Ten or so people waited for us to move him onto their stretcher so they could take over. I gave the report.

"Seventy-six-year-old male, conscious at 11:15, found by family not breathing at 11:30. CPR started at 11:35. Twenty-gauge IV in left AC at 1140, epi at 1141, atropine at 1143, remained pulseless and asystolic. History of stroke five years ago and Alzheimer's."

The hospital team took over, we backed out. Another round of epi and atropine, then other meds, five minutes later I heard the attending:

"I've got a pulse."

Ten minutes later he was breathing on his own, blood pressure rising.

An hour later he was still with us. It's ten hours later and he is still with us.

Regardless of our beliefs or feelings, we have a job to do. Once resuscitation efforts are started, training and experience takes over, everybody gives their best effort, and a power higher than us decides the outcome.

His son and granddaughter were at his side the last time I looked. Everybody was at peace.

Bad Dog

All day, nothin' to do, think I'll lay on this couch, now I'll take a nap, now I'll look out the window, nobody home, can't wait. Boy it's hot up here, when are they coming home? Think I'll take a nap, look out the window, drink some water, get on the couch, where are they?

Nothin' to do, take a nap, look out the window, water's gone, have to pee, better not do it here, look out the window, soon I hope, when are they coming home? Getting dark, I'm hungry, sit on the couch take a nap, forget I'm hungry, can't wait, is that them?

Not yet, gotta pee bad, no water in my bowl, lay on the couch, look out the window, take a nap, lay on the couch . . . wait, what's that?

Oh boy, here they are, come on dad, hurry up, I gotta pee, oh boy, finally I hate to be alone, come on dad, I've been good all day, it's hot up here, let me out, I'm dying up here, please hurry. Closer now, the door's opening, oh boy, they're home!

Ouch! Why did he do that? Ouch! Come on, dad, cut it out. I know that smell, oh no, here comes another one. Ouch! That hurts. I get it, you're the alpha male, I'm the dog. Ouch, jeez, I just had to pee soo bad, Ouch! For God's sake, man . . . Ouch . . .

One more and I'm going to lose it . . . Ouch!

The family pet attacked his owners tonight. A man and his wife had been out drinking. When they got home after being gone all day the man started teasing his dog. He had him since he was a puppy, seven years ago. He couldn't figure out why his dog snapped. I covered his hand that had been nearly bitten in half and put a trauma dressing on his other arm; bone, muscle, and tendons were showing before it was dressed. We needed another rescue for his wife. And animal control to take the dog away.

He'll be put down by week's end.

Adorable

A six-, seven-, and twenty-five-year-old just lit up the back of Rescue 3 like nobody's business. Talasia had a fever. Her sister Shalasia held her hand all the way out of the apartment in the middle of the projects and to the hospital. Their mom looked just like them, only older. They wore matching pajamas and matching sandals. The rescue fascinated them; they seemed particularly fond of the lights.

Would I have called 911 at one in the morning to take my seven-year-old to the ER for a fever of 102 degrees? Hell no! But they were adorable, and being able to see that instead of being angry sometimes makes all the difference.

Cooked
WARNING

Lieutenant Morse has swallowed a bitter pill.

Take an extremely overweight middle-aged non-English-speaking woman, add twelve prescription medications, mix one ridiculously expensive king-sized bed in a government-subsidized apartment, three parts fawning non-English-speaking relatives, a huge helping of drama, a pinch of vomit, and two sets of stairs and you will get a person who "can't move" until she sees the stair chair miraculously appear at the foot of her bed, then is able to drag herself from the previously mentioned king-sized bed in the government-subsidized apartment and plant herself into the chair, then let herself be carried down the previously mentioned two flights of stairs into an ambulance that carts her to a world-class emergency room where she will be given thousands of dollars worth of tests to get to the bottom of her abdominal pain, which will go away on its own if given a chance.

Mix well. Bake in the back of the rescue until done. Repeat five times after midnight.

The Lion and the Mule

My friend Dave had a little setback. He's in New London Hospital recovering from surgery on the same weekend three of his daughters are moving into two different colleges.

Enter the mule.

I'm actually having a ball, getting to know the girls a little better and helping a friend in need. On the way here I ran into the funeral procession for Senator Ted Kennedy. People stood on roadways and overpasses during torrential downpours and strong winds to pay their respects to the "Liberal Lion" as he passed. I hadn't really given his death much thought and was moved much more than I ever expected by the outpouring of grief. As I drove I couldn't stop the internal movie from playing. I was born the year JFK was assassinated, seven or so when Robert was killed. The Kennedys have been a big part of my surroundings since I can remember.

As I passed through Manchester I said a silent hello to my friend Walt, paid a silent respect to Ted, and kept on trucking.

Not Me

"What happened to you?"

He stood by the side of the road, his scalp nearly torn from his head, blood cascading down his face, a few fingers appeared broken along with his nose.

"I got hit by a car."

The woman who stood by him, a pretty twenty-five-year-old, shivered as the warm night air blew down Atwells Avenue toward Olneyville. She was confused, maybe intoxicated, I couldn't tell. Another rescue was called while I treated the allegedly struck pedestrian.

"Everybody says you were driving the car that took out two poles and a tree and landed on its roof."

"I was hit by a car."

"Whatever."

Three blocks up the road emergency crews were busy cleaning up the wake of the "pedestrian struck," drunken tour of the neighborhood. An expensive car lie on its side, three of the five occupants being transported to the trauma rooms. The driver had already been identified as the guy now boarded and collared in my truck.

"So, what happened?"

"I told you, I got hit by a car."

"Everybody else is telling me you were driving the car that nearly killed four people and the driver."

"Wasn't me."

We started a few IVs, started him on O2, stopped the blood loss, the bottoms of my shoes were covered, and took him in. At the hospital the cops waited. I told them what I knew, the guy continued to deny any responsibility. It really was pathetic.

I am in no way condoning intoxicated driving, but people do it all the time. Most get away with it, wake up the next day, and do it all over again. Some get caught, weaving between the lines or whatever, others crash their vehicles into trees or drive off the road, others go up on ramps the wrong way and kill innocent people. A few go to prison for the same crime a big part of the population is guilty of at one time or another but was fortunate enough to get away with. Some die.

Others are fortunate enough to get behind the wheel, full of arrogance, put four other people's lives in jeopardy and drive like an idiot with zero regard for anybody but themselves, and take out a tree and a pole, flip the car, nearly have their head removed but walk away.

The police left the hospital. I asked if they were going to lock the guy up when he was released from the hospital.

"We're not pressing charges, no evidence."

If you must drive drunk, do it in Providence.

Fill the Boot

We helped him out of his wheelchair, onto the stretcher, and into the back of Rescue 1. His mom stepped in and sat on the bench seat.

"What's your name, buddy," I asked.

"David," answered Mom and David.

"What's wrong?"

"Nothing." (David)

"His stomach hurts." (Mom)

I moved from the captain's chair and sat next to David's mom, directly across from him.

"What's wrong, David?"

"I haven't gone to the bathroom in three days." His dark skin actually turned red.

Strange how thirteen-year-old boys have difficulty telling strangers about private matters.

"You know, David, everybody shits."

He laughed and relaxed a little.

"Not me."

"Why are you in that wheelchair?" I asked.

"Muscular dystrophy."

He was born with it. Up until a year ago everything was fine, then the pain and weakness set in. There is no cure. He will die from his disease, long before he should.

"It's not that bad," he said and smiled at his mom, who was near tears.

This weekend, do us all a favor, and "Fill the Boot."

Labor Day

I grew up in a union household. My father belonged to the IBEW until he was promoted and took a job in management, taking with him the morality and ethics of his union membership. I remember my uncle, Bill, proudly wearing his Teamsters cap. Uncle Ron was a Warwick cop. Brian was president of his union at Rhode Island College. We would spend summer days at their homes, surrounded by family, the American flag always flying, either on a flagpole or attached to the house, the red, white, and blue proudly displayed.

Modest homes meticulously kept, hard work, and an ability to enjoy the fruits of their labor and share them with friends and family was all they wanted. Uncle Bill was a World War II vet, my father a Navy signalman during the Korean War. Brian served in the Air Force during the Vietnam War. They lived, and live, good, honest lives, are fiercely proud of their country, and fought for the freedoms we now enjoy. Union members. Not everybody in my family, but those I remember most.

My brother, Bob, just returned from Iraq. Five hundred days. Another union man. Myself, a firefighter in Providence. Union. We are living in the shadow of our uncles and father, and it is my belief we have made them proud.

Some of our union leaders have let us down, just as some of our elected officials have let us down. Politics is a cutthroat business, and like it or not, everything is political. Those that have risen to the top of our ranks thrive in that arena; most of us would rather do our jobs, do them well, and live our lives. We need people in positions of power for us to do that.

Relentless media attacks have insulated the union ranks. An us-against-them attitude prevails. Gone are the days when a union worked with management in a respectful, productive atmosphere. Maybe that never existed; I don't know. Gold-plated benefits, feeding at the public trough, picking our pockets, and on and on. Socialists, communists, serving the weak, protecting the incompetent—enough already!

The governor of the state of Rhode Island has gone to the national airwaves to justify his decision to shut down state government for twelve days this year. State revenues are down as our tourist industry bears the weight of a struggling economy. The state coffers are empty. Aid to cities and towns are on the chopping block as well.

Again, union members are asked to give "their share" back to the community. The taxpayers need a break, the logic goes, the unions must make concessions. "It's only fair."

How is it "fair" that a segment of the population makes contractual concessions for years, gives back here and there and everywhere, then takes twelve days off without pay? If every adult in Rhode Island were to write a check equal to what municipal union members have already given back, our budget problems would be over.

I hereby relinquish my soapbox for the rest of the day, you may go in peace. Thanks for listening. Enjoy the weekend; it's going to be a beauty here in Rhode Island.

Black Clouds

We drove past the building where a man jumped to his death yesterday. I looked at the place, counted the floors and focused on the window I thought to be the one he jumped out of. I played it over in my mind, just as Zack told the story to me yesterday, minutes after he brought the patient, still breathing then, into the trauma room.

"We got there first," Zack explained, "the people in the lobby told me his wife had him but couldn't hold on much longer."

"Where were the cops?" I asked.

"Not there yet, I went alone. As soon as I opened the door to the apartment he went nuts, started throwing things at me, bottles, chairs, anything he could get his hands on."

"What did you do?"

"I had to back out. He wasn't attacking his wife, but I set him off. The window was open, I didn't think he would jump . . ."

The incident was twenty minutes old at this time. Not enough time to sort things out, the emotions too raw. Zack runs Rescue 4, located downtown on the same group as me. We've worked together for nearly eight years now. They call people like me and Zack "Black Clouds." We just seem to get a lot of the horrible calls.

"He could have taken you with him," I said, bringing Zack back.

"I could have stopped him."

And so it goes, another piece taken from the armor of one of the best rescue guys in Providence.

Humbled

"She's out of control."

Five feet tall, one hundred pounds soaking wet, beautiful and twenty-five, how bad could it be? She had tried to go to a popular nightclub in the Silver Lake section of Providence. Showed her money, hugged the bouncer, and staggered in the doorway. They wouldn't let her in. She threw her cell phone and thirty bucks at the bouncer, started screaming. Security got involved, couldn't control her, and called for police and rescue. We arrived before the cops. She was all over the security guard at this time, hugging him, all lovey-dovey.

"She's all yours," he said.

"I'll handle this," I said to Ben, my partner for the night. "I speak the language of love."

I figured my *Sesame Street* Spanish, boyish good looks, and uniform would be all I needed to tame this wild Spanish dynamo. The Spanish-speaking security guard looked doubtful. Ben shrugged and stood to the side.

"What are they saying, anyway?" I asked Ben, who is fluent in Spanish.

"He's telling her she's too drunk to enter, she says she wants to party, he says she can party tomorrow, she wants to stay."

"I'm all over this."

"Hola, mami," I said, big smile on my face. "Estas buena mama sota!"

I think I said, "Hello, lady, you look very beautiful." She looked me in the eye, got all silent for a moment, broke free from the security guard, and opened a full assault on the boyishly charming Spanish-speaking idiot who stood in front of her. Fortunately, my catlike reflexes are still intact; I sidestepped a few punches, dodged the spit, stepped away from the kicks, and ran away.

"Stupid ugly American!" she shouted as Ben grabbed her and kept her away from me.

"I thought you didn't speak English," I said, keeping my distance.

"Want me to take over?" asked Ben.

Within a minute he had her on the stretcher, calm as can be and cooperating. She was getting very friendly; I called for assistance. It's never a good idea to transport a single intoxicated aggressive female alone in the back of a rescue.

"Rescue 2 to fire alarm, transporting an intoxicated female to Rhode Island Hospital, mileage 216112."

"Message received Rescue 2, to Rhode Island."

I left the scene, took what I thought to be a shortcut through the neighborhood, and promptly got lost in the maze. Two miles later I reappeared on the main road, found the highway, and delivered our prize to the ER.

I transmitted our ending mileage to fire alarm and hid in the front while the guys finished the job.

If nothing else, things like this keep me humble!

Connected

The old lady on the stretcher slipped in and out of consciousness as we rode toward the hospital. Her daughter leaned over from the bench seat, stroking her mother's forehead and holding her hand. I felt like an intruder, sitting behind them in the captain's seat, filling out the report, but they didn't seem to mind my presence, their bond stronger than anything I ever felt.

The lady in the stretcher was nearing the end of her life, eighty-one years old and not in the best of health. This would be her third trip to the hospital this month; she has been passing out and falling for no reason. Her daughter looked intently into her mother's eyes as we rode. Letting a parent go is never easy; my own mother suffered a major stroke at age fifty-six and lingered for another nine years in a nursing home, never regaining her sense of self.

I stopped writing and watched the two interact. It occurred to me that the twenty-five or so years that were stolen from my mother and me could have been time to heal old wounds, get to know each other, and enter into a more adult relationship. I envied the opportunity these two had but was happy for them as well.

An hour earlier I took another elderly person from his home, also accompanied by a daughter. They too had that special bond. She helped him walk to the rescue; he insisted even though his weakened legs barely held him up. The daughter was able to take care of the father now, and he let her, grateful for the assistance.

My own father died when I was twenty-eight. I had barely grown up, tried to be there for him during his yearlong battle with cancer, and did the best I could, but I now know that at twenty-eight the best I could do wasn't nearly as good as I could do now that I've lived and experienced life for twenty more years. Father and daughter rode together in my truck, comfortable in each other's presence, as I sat alone behind them.

Funny what runs through your mind when you least expect it. Although fall is my favorite time of year, the evidence of our mortality must sink in to my subconscious mind as flowers die, leaves get tired, and days get shorter. It isn't a bad thing, it actually makes me appreciate the time I have here and now and puts a little urgency in the way I handle my relationships with the people who mean the world to me.

Zack just called, somebody got murdered in front of Crossroads. Nothing he could do this time, just declare the man dead and move on to the next one. The city had been quiet for an hour or two, and then something happened. I swear a pulse or something unseen permeates the atmosphere at times and drives people to do insane things. As Zack leaned over a man who had his head split open with a machete, I sat in the back of Rescue 1 on the way to Miriam with a man who had just tried to kill himself with a knife, and Theresa and John at Rescue 5 treated another suicidal knife-wielding patient.

Six hours to go. Except for a few hours I've been here since Friday, dozens of calls, a few emergencies, little sleep.

9/11

The plan was to go to the beach and enjoy one of the last brilliant days of summer. Instead, we sat in front of the TV, shaking our heads when we could move them, calling friends and family and just feeling numb. An eerie silence smothered my neighborhood as the day progressed, the crystal clear air and eighty degree temperature seeming to mock the dismal mood that permeated my surroundings. The state airport half a mile away might as well have been a desert, nothing stirred, no low hum of planes taxiing, no roar of jet engines whining before the roar of takeoff, no noise, no movement, nothing but the sound of bugs and birds and the occasional car as it passed on the main road, half a mile away.

When I could, I tore myself away from the television screen; the first tower had fallen, followed by the second some time later. The time between is lost to me, my memories flash them collapsing in quick succession.

"We just lost hundreds of firefighters," I said to my wife as we watched the tragedy unfold.

"Surely they weren't still inside," she replied, horror and emotion choking the words.

"They were."

Some things you just know.

I stood in the doorway of my garage, listening to the silence, hoping for the roar of a plane taking off, an F-16, a B-52, a Blackhawk . . . anything as long as it was headed over there, where, I had no idea but felt certain Washington knew, but the same deafening silence filled the quiet streets. I crossed my arms, shook my head, and stood there, unable to move.

In the corner, leaning against a bunch of hockey sticks and a broom, was my salvation. I walked closer, stood there for a moment, really seeing it for the first time, even though I put it out every Fourth of July, Memorial and Veterans Days, and some others if I remembered. I was only paralyzed for a moment, then took action. It was a tiny bit of energy expelled on my part, a few steps, grasping the pole, unfurling the flag, putting it into the porcelain holder I had screwed into my garage years before, and stepping back. Almost magically a breeze, one of the very few that blew that day, pushed past my home, opening the flag in its full glory, waving, and then resting. That small act made me feel a lot better about things and I silently thanked those who have fought and died so that I had the opportunity to perform my private ceremony, thus mourning the lost and rekindling my patriotic spirit that had lay dormant for years.

Later that day, I left for work, still stunned and shell-shocked, my view of the world changed forever. I said goodbye to Cheryl, lingering a little longer than usual, both of us realizing how precious our lives really are. In a daze I drove the usual route, past the homes, through Pawtuxet Village, into Cranston, eventually arriving in Providence.

Of all the things about that day I will "Never Forget," the hundreds of American flags that magically appeared along my route remain the most vivid. On doorways, utility poles, storefronts, from car windows, everywhere I could see the red, white, and blue flew proudly.

The best part of it all is nobody told us to do it, it hadn't become fashionable yet, it just was. There were a lot of private ceremonies going on that day. I didn't know it but I was never alone when I stood in front of my garage and planted the flag proudly on my home.

I will "Never Forget" those that perished that day, especially the firefighters, EMTs, and police officers who answered the call for help.

And as my ride to work on September 11, 2001, showed me, neither will anybody else.

Cramps

"Rescue 1, respond to the soccer field for a twenty-one-year-old male laying in a silver van complaining of leg cramps."

"Leg cramps?" I said to myself.

"Laying in a van?" I said to myself.

"Rescue 1 responding," I said into the radio.

Our patient was indeed lying on the back seat of the college's athletic transport van, motor idling, waiting for the "paramedics" to administer an IV and fluids to alleviate the cramping legs.

"He needs an IV right away," said the athletic trainer, a tiny woman who knelt on the floor of the van massaging the player's legs.

"He's already getting what he needs." I couldn't help myself.

"He played 110 minutes, he's dehydrated," she said, rubbing his calves.

"I've worked 110 hours, I'm dehydrated." Again, I couldn't help myself.

Ryan brought the stretcher over to the side door of the van, the player couldn't move. We got a backboard to make our lives easier and got him into the rescue.

"We're taking him to the hospital," I told the trainer.

"He just needs IV fluids, can't you just do it here?"

People honestly believe that the city of Providence has unlimited resources, can dispatch an advanced life support rescue to a soccer field to administer IV fluids to a soccer player while true emergencies are tended to by all the other rescues that are sitting around waiting for something to do. As I tended to our patient, the people at fire alarm were on the phone trying to find rescues from neighboring communities to answer the calls that keep on coming.

We started an IV and headed toward the ER. The trainer came with us, followed by the van. They were not happy with our response. Neither was I.

Where's Home?

They looked alike, maybe father and son, maybe brothers, I couldn't tell. Turns out they weren't related, just good friends. Veterans of the Iraq War. The older guy had called us to take care of his friend, a thirty-year-old guy suffering from PTSD.

They stood as we approached, not sure what the future held. I opened the passenger door and walked toward them, also unsure what to expect. Two guys sitting on the steps of an old building in Roger Williams Park at three o'clock on a Sunday afternoon could need a number of things, usually detox.

"Did you guys call 911?"

The younger of the two looked down. He had been crying. His friend explained.

"I've been talking to him all day but he can't stop crying. I think he wants to kill himself."

The young guy looked miserable. I helped him into the rescue, his friend walked away without saying goodbye.

"What's going on?" I asked.

He handed me his VA card.

"I can't keep it together. Nothing works. I can't keep a job, I haven't seen my daughter, I just want to go home."

"Where is home?"

"North Carolina."

He showed me his shoulder, the scars from small arms fire recently healed. They put the body back together; the mind is slow to follow. During the ten-minute ride to the VA I learned a lot about him; sometimes strangers have a way of communicating that is more intimate than the closest of friends. It's safer talking to people you don't know and probably will never see again.

He did most of the talking, he needed somebody to listen. His story was all too familiar. Once discharged from active service, the world outside the military isn't always the kindest place. The Northeast isn't always the kindest place. Iraq definitely wasn't the kindest place.

I told him it's okay to get on with his life. His emotional wounds would never fully heal, but a good life was possible in spite of what he had survived. Medication, therapy, and communicating would help, and there is nothing wrong with any of those things, just tools, or in his view weapons to be used against the potentially deadly enemy he faced.

I'm not sure if he heard me, or remembered anything I said, but I felt a lot better knowing I was able to make our short time together tolerable for him, at least for a little while.

I walked with him into the VA. Without looking up from her computer screen the secretary asked, "Last four."

He told her. She put the last four numbers of his Social Security number into the system and told him to take a seat.

False Alarm

"Rescue 1 and Engine 10, respond to 12 Broad Street for an infant not breathing."

It's a long ride, even at full speed, in the middle of the night, lights and sirens blaring through the empty streets. A call for an infant not breathing is a nightmare. Ghosts of prior fatalities, the littlest ones, climb on board and take the ride with us, their blue faces and eerily cold, stiff bodies right there in the front of the cab, keeping us company. Protocols, procedures, and a plan how best to deal with distraught parents make room for the memories as the destination nears.

The fire company arrives first, their own ghosts following them to the third floor. They are rushing, one after the other, running up the steps toward their patient. The rescue stops in front of the house, we get out and follow.

I'm sorry if we weren't all laughter and smiles when we saw your beautiful daughter sitting on your lap, breathing normally, perhaps a little sniffle, fully dressed and waiting for a ride to the ER for free medication. Sorry if we disturbed your sense of entitlement when the fire guys voiced their displeasure at your inability to communicate. Sorry that learning to speak the language of your new country is low on your list of priorities.

Next time get your story straight before setting things in motion. Or find somebody who can.

Better

Nestled between free rides to the hospital for routine medical care an occasional gem slips through.

"My heart is racing."

I put her on the monitor. 180. Racing indeed. We started an IV, put her on oxygen, and instructed her to "bear down." Nothing worked. I got 6 mg of adenosine ready, John filled a 20 ml syringe with normal saline.

"You're going to feel strange," I said to her. She nodded her head. I attached the medication to the IV line, looked at John, pinched the line, and pushed. John followed immediately with the flush.

Her rhythm slowed, down to 140, but shot back up.

"We're going to try that again."

She closed her eyes and waited. We repeated the procedure. I waited for the flat line but it never appeared, just a slow, steady sinus rhythm. It leveled off at 100.

"How do you feel?"

"Better."

Making people feel better. That is what it's all about.

Taxi 1

Anybody who has worked for more than a few years in EMS is well aware of the socialist tendency of our services. As the debate in Washington rages on, the left supporting health care reform, the right satisfied with the status quo, we continue to provide "free" transportation for marginally ill people to the nation's emergency rooms.

I often wonder how things have gotten so out of control. People call 911 for a ride to the ER while their family waits, driveway full of cars, then follow us to the hospital. Once we arrive at their home, more often than not, the patient informs us of his or her hospital of choice, and then is surprised and indignant when I inform him or her I'll gladly take them to the closest hospital to treat their emergency; if they need to get to the hospital of choice they will have to arrange other transportation.

A lot of people find this disturbing. "Just do your job," I've heard more than once.

My job, I think, is to respond to emergencies, and treat and transport seriously ill people to the appropriate medical facility. It is not, at least for the time being, a taxi service.

What is next? A three-digit phone call for free rides to the grocery store because a person is hungry?

In case you are considering this post more grumbling by a disgruntled employee, consider this litany of nonsense from the weekend:

Difficulty swallowing (no allergic reaction).

Ten-year-old "out of control."

Emotional twenty-four-year-old male who broke up with his boyfriend.

Twenty-two-year-old female with a tooth infection.

Seventy-year-old who needs medication refilled.

Intoxicated male in bed at home seeking detox.

Blood pressure needs to be "checked."

MVA in parking lot, zero damage, barely moving vehicles, three occupants boarded and collared, transported to the ER.

Two-year-old female with a fever of 101.

The patent's insurance company or, in most cases here, the government is billed anywhere from $350 to more than $1,000 depending on the length of the ride and treatment.

There has to be a better way.

Rear Window

I'd been to the house a few times, saw the layout, and visualized how we would get her out when she died. I hoped it would be peacefully, in her sleep. Then, the coroner could come, or the funeral home people and remove her from her home with some dignity. Sadly, that was not the case.

At 0930 we received the call: a woman not breathing. I knew the address was familiar, when we approached the mental images flooded into my mind. A wheelchair. An obese woman. A tracheotomy and colostomy bag. Diabetic supplies, needles, insulin bottles, blood glucose monitors, cotton balls, donuts. The doorway, narrow. The family, equally as large, equally in denial, empty pizza boxes, candy, everything that shouldn't be but was.

The guys from Engine 11 had started CPR in the doorway. I struggled over the patient, checked the defibrillator pads, had them halt CPR, waited for the machine to do its job.

No Shock Advised.

CPR continued, a backboard was brought into the apartment, she was rolled on her side and strapped down, chest compressions done to the best of our ability throughout, airway maintained, IVs attempted. I had my new partner, Ryan, get the intubation equipment prepared and the back of the truck ready as we carried her out. The stretcher groaned, but held.

Inside the truck, daughter standing outside, lost, crying, afraid. I closed the door, she stared at the truck, unable to move. The intubation attempt was unsuccessful, IV access not obtained. All we could do was CPR and rapid transport.

I looked out the rear window, the solitary figure of a girl, the same size as her dying mother, filled the opening at first, but shrank the further we travelled, until she disappeared.

We tried. All the way to the ER, six IV attempts failed. When there is no pump to fill the veins other than chest compressions done in back of a speeding truck, the chance of a successful stick is minimal. Another ET attempt failed, this time my own. I visualized the vocal cords, had everything in place but the tube just wouldn't advance.

"Keep doing CPR, try to keep the airway open and save whatever brain cells she has in case they revive her."

It was akin to surrender but there is little we can do without proper IV access or a tube to administer meds. The ride was over before I knew it, the patient delivered to the medical team that had assembled. I gave the story to the attending, apologizing for the lack of IV or tube. He put a hand on my shoulder, looked me in the eye, looked at the patient, and said we did a good job.

Somehow, they got a heartbeat. She was on a respirator when I walked out. I saw her daughter in the distance, in front of the family services office. For a moment I considered walking the long corridor and offering some comfort, but it just seemed too far.

Speak Up!
"WHAT?"

"What are you doing down there?"

"SPEAK UP!"

I leaned closer to her ear.

"I SAID, WHAT ARE YOU DOING DOWN THERE?"

"WATCHING THE TELEVISION!"

There was no TV in the room, just another elderly patient suffering from dementia. Ethel was on her back, a four-inch laceration over her left eye, dried blood all over her face.

Bruising had already begun, the sickly yellow color a sharp contrast to her milky white skin.

"We're going to take you to the hospital," I said as the guys got the backboard and collar ready.

"I'M IN THE HOSPITAL!" she said.

"Well, we're taking you to a different hospital then."

"GOOD! THE FOOD HERE IS LOUSY!"

Without further ado we left the place. I looked at the interagency report on the way to the ER. She had been living at the same place for five years. Dementia is difficult for family and friends; I'm not sure how bad it is for the patients.

Some People

A guy's wife has had four seizures since midnight. It's 4:00 a.m. She's sitting in a chair in their living room, unaware. We get the stair chair ready and carry her out of their home and into the rescue.

"She goes to Miriam."

"She's having seizures. The closest hospital is Rhode Island, we'll take her there."

"She goes to Miriam."

"Not tonight."

The ride is uncomfortable. He glares at me all the way. She begins to seize. He looks at me as though I caused this. For some unknown reason I feel the need to explain the situation to him. Miriam is ten minutes away, Rhode Island three. I'm sure we would make it to Miriam without any harm to the patient, but sometimes you have to go on principle. Rhode Island and Miriam are one. The same doctors, the same record-keeping system, the same company. There was no wait at either facility at this hour.

It's odd, how a person can be angry at somebody who rushes to their house in the middle of the night, carries their wife out the door, onto a stretcher and into a rescue, gives her oxygen, starts an IV, assesses her vital signs, administers medication to help with the seizure, and gets her to a world-class hospital in less than thirty minutes from the time he made the call.

I love this job, and get paid well to do it, but some people . . .

Last Act

How many people are affected by every call we go on? Obviously, the people making the 911 call, then the dispatchers, then us, then the people who hear the sirens and see the lights, and get out of the way, or not. Neighbors, friends, family: everybody who sees a fire truck, police cruiser, or ambulance pull up at somebody's house can't help but be curious.

It's like a ripple in the universe; I wonder how far it goes. When the outcome is positive, does the energy go forward and add to the general flow of things, and if so, when things go badly does that change the tide for everybody involved, no matter how small a part?

A few years ago I realized how important my role in all of this is. When I arrive on scene at an emergency, every move I make is embedded into the memory of the people who called for help. It may be subconsciously, but the experience lingers.

Years pass. The memory fades. Some things stand out. The time the ambulance people helped dad when he fell. When Mom crashed her car on 95, the firemen were so nice. They helped the baby when she swallowed a marble. They tried their hardest to get Grandma back but it was just her time to die.

It is an enormous responsibility, one not to be taken lightly. For generations people will talk about us when they get together. How we act lives long after the act itself is over.

Falling

A kid fell off the escalator at the Providence Place Mall Saturday night. Adam, my once and future partner, was first on scene. He told me the worst part for him is rolling the patient and seeing the face for the first time. Often, it is the face of death.

A while ago I was on scene at the same mall on the same lower level landing spot with the same situation. This time it was a girl, twenty-three years old, one in the morning, dressed for a night out with her fiancé. Her earrings survived the forty-foot fall off the side of the escalator, they were still attached, looking strangely out of place nestled in the blood-soaked hair. Silver hoops, I recall, reflecting the fluorescent lights three floors above. She must have landed on the back of her head, it felt like applesauce when I reached my hand back there to lift it and place the cervical collar. Her eyes were closed. I lifted the lids and shined my light into them. Fixed and dilated. A ladder company was there to assist, I stepped back and watched as they placed her on the spine board and loaded her onto the stretcher.

"Is she alright?" asked a guy about her age who stood nearby.

What do you say? We are trained to tell family and friends generic information, "we're doing all we can," things like that.

A Spider-Man doll lay on the floor, a few feet from the pool of blood that had formed around her head. She had won it at the nightclub they spent the night at, celebrating both her birthday and her graduation from the local junior college. She had planned on giving it to her four-year-old in the morning, he loved Spider-Man.

I held her head in my left hand, the collar giving me some support as we rode to the ER, bagging her with my right. I let her eyes remain closed as we cut off her outfit, so carefully put on only hours before, and covered her with a sheet. There were more injuries, but no sense treating them. She was gone.

I often wonder if I should have ended my involvement there, passed her off to the people at the ER and moved on. Instead, I talked with her fiancé, asked about who she was, where she came from. He needed to talk, I needed to listen. Now, instead of another memory embedded deep in my subconscious, I have a vivid recollection of the event, and to this day need to catch my breath every time I walk past the spot she fell; the same spot that may or may not hold the same emotional impact for Adam.

One Hand Pizza

It takes a lot to get a rise out of old Lieutenant Morse. Lacerations, fractures, amputations, eviscerations—I've seen it all. Not impressed with the little scrapes and bruises some people just can't handle.

Take a simple burn, for instance. Some moron put his pizza box and all into the 350-degree oven to keep it warm while he shut down the house. Lights off, shades drawn, drinks made, movie ready, maybe five minutes.

At pizza time he reached into the oven, grasped the cardboard box firmly in his hands, and headed toward the table. Ignoring the pain he felt when he hoisted the box from the hot oven, "there is no possible way a cardboard box could be this hot," he reasoned, "surely the box would ignite." He walked the twenty feet, refusing to put the box down.

Ten seconds later, after squealing like a little bitch and flinging the cursed box and all its contents onto the table, Mrs. Lieutenant Morse appeared with the bottle of aloe vera, washed the hot oil from his red hand, and put him to bed, where he ate pizza one-handed.

Timeout

Rescuing Providence? How about rescuing the guy who says he's rescuing Providence? Looks like ole Lieutenant Morse will be playing patient for a while. I finally took recurring back pain seriously and had an MRI, turns out things aren't so great back there. My doctor asked if there are any supervisory positions on Rescue 1. After I stopped giggling I realized she was serious.

I have a surgical consult next week and extensive PT in the meantime.

Some advice from an old coot if you care to listen: Enjoy each day you are on the trucks, learn something about yourself and how better to treat every patient that crosses your path. Appreciate the fact that what you do, though seemingly thankless and mundane at times, is without a doubt one of, if not the most important and worthy professions out there.

Your next lift could be your last. It happens fast, one day you're the king of the world, limitless possibilities and things to blog about, the next your future is uncertain, and your back hurts like hell.

Free Ride

Physical therapy is going well, those people are truly amazing. I always heard it is a difficult program, now I know why. I described my injury to the therapist; he had me do a series of movements, each one taking pressure off of my squished discs. I found it miraculous how simple movements could be so effective. If I keep doing the exercises, things should be back in place before long.

While there I was talking to a guy about an experience he and his wife had over the weekend. She had some lower abdominal pain and went to the ER at Women and Infants Hospital. They drove there, their car was right outside. The doctor at the ER decided the patient should be medically cleared at a regular emergency facility rather than one specializing in maternity and such and wanted them to go to Rhode Island Hospital, which is on the same campus and actually connected by an underground tunnel.

"I'll call the Providence Fire Department," he told them. "They'll send a rescue."

"Our car is right outside," the guy told him.

"It's a liability issue," replied the doctor.

So, there you have it. The medical community is as clueless as the rest of the population who abuse the 911 system on a daily basis. I can hardly wait for whatever health care reform comes out of Washington. Something tells me I'll be driving people to physical therapy appointments, at taxpayer expense.

When I Am King

Official Decree from the King

1. I hereby decree that any person or persons within a sixty (60) mile radius of Boston wearing a New York Yankees cap or any other New York Yankees paraphernalia, including but not limited to bumper stickers, banners, flags, or statues, be subject to a Yankee Facts test to ensure their loyalty to the team they so proudly display on their person, vehicle, and home.

2. Persons failing Yankee Facts test mentioned in paragraph 1 will be incarcerated until such time they agree to never again display New York Yankee items in the heart of Red Sox Nation.

3. Yankee Facts test mentioned in paragraph 1 will have a sliding scale of difficulty, increasing in difficulty starting further from Boston toward points inward.

4. Upon release from prison, buses will be provided to all Yankee-wearing, test-failing, shit-stirring New York

wannabes from HERE to THERE, where you will be deposited in the heart of Yankee country with the rest of the Yankee fans. Construction of a giant wall will begin, at Steinbrenner's expense, to keep said "fans" penned in.

5. All surrendered Yankee paraphernalia will be collected and burned in Town Square, where music, food, and moonlight dancing will be provided to all pitchfork-wielding townspeople.

So it is written, so it shall be done! **No Hugs!**
What is up with all this handshake huggy stuff all the young guys are doing now? Every time I go to shake somebody's hand who happens to be under thirty, they drag me in and give me a hug. Don't like it. Nothing personal, but I like my space. My brother, the Iraq War veteran, correctional officer, all-around tough guy and I have been through fistfights, rock fights, a knife fight or two, and a couple of gunfights—never hugged. Children have been born, homes bought, parents died, kids graduated, milestone after milestone and we never hugged. The last time we touched anything other than our right hands was our last episode of kung fu, Ali-Frazier wrestling when we were twelve and ten. I love the man, and am not afraid to say it—I'd take a bullet for him—but NO HUGS!

From here on, if anybody attempts to hug me during a handshake, I will be forced to assume I'm being brought close for something deadly, a shiv attack or worse, and respond with deadly force of my own. The ancient Babylonians started the handshake as a means of holding their enemies hand to avert an attack. That's when men were men, no hugging allowed. I like it that way, nice and simple.

If you feel an overwhelming desire to hug while greeting, substitutes are acceptable. Wives, girlfriends, and hot mothers will do.

Authority

I found myself in the hot seat at Brown University last night, answering questions from students considering a career in medicine. One of the students, Brita Larson, invited me to talk with the class in an informal setting about my opinions and experience with emergency medical services.

Considering I am my favorite subject, I couldn't refuse. The students were great and seemed genuinely interested in what I had to say. I've been writing my thoughts and opinions for so long it was a welcome change to talk with people and be able to immediately see their reactions to what I had to say. Writing is much safer, I learned. It is easy to write something, let it sit for a while, then reread it and change things that don't sound quite right. Talking is on the record, then and there, no looking back. I found myself questioning some of my own opinions about poverty, lifestyle, and the need for reform in our "industry" after the class. I've never been one to hold back my ideas, it's just that nobody really listens to idle conversation. These kids did listen, and looked to me as an authority and expert in my field, and it occurred to me halfway through that I actually am.

Thank you, Brita and the rest of the class, for welcoming me into your world for a little while. I hope you enjoyed the hour as much as I did.

Healing

Funny thing about back problems: everybody seems to have one. Whenever I tell somebody I'm recuperating from a back injury I get the usual, "Don't I know it, my back *kills*!"

In all fairness, I'm guilty of the same. Whenever somebody tells me about their aching back I'm the first to chime in with "you don't know the half of it!"

So, anyway, while my back continues to improve I've been keeping busy. I actually have no idea how I ever found time to work. I do have to do things more slowly and actually think before I move, or a big surprise is in store. I still can't get used to being on half speed.

If nothing else I've learned some humility. As some of you may know, my wife is battling multiple sclerosis. Walking underwater with a limp is a good way to describe how she gets around; it really is quite difficult. Simple things I take for granted, such as rolling over in bed, are a monumental task for her. While I've never taken her condition lightly, I never really understood the frustration of wanting to do something but being unable. That is the worst, waiting for somebody to help. I think I know a tenth of what she feels now.

So, that is my silver lining for today. Crummy silver lining, I know, but it's all I've got.

I'd like to thank everybody who still stops by here, I really appreciate it. I know not much is happening, and there is a ton of other things to occupy your time, so THANK YOU! I think I'm an egomaniac, I actually get quite sad if nobody is paying attention to me.

Hard Landing

My friend Ryan is twenty-three. He's been a Providence firefighter for about a year. When Adam left the rescue for Engine 7 on North Main Street, Ryan took over. We had only worked together for a month or so when I injured my back, but in that short span of time I learned we have a lot in common: love for the job, compassion for our patients, and the desire to do the best job we can.

Two days ago, a man ripped off his seat belt and slammed his car into a bridge abutment as his girlfriend sat in the passenger seat. We will probably never know what caused him to do it, only that he did. When the crash didn't kill him he ran from the car, onto an overpass, and jumped into the northbound lanes of Interstate 95 North. Four cars hit him.

Ryan and Dave were first on scene. It should have been me and Ryan, and for Ryan's sake I wish it was. Nothing against Dave, he is more than capable, but at incidents like these it helps to be with your regular partner. The scene Ryan described to me as he drove home from work, alone in his truck for the first time since the incident, was horrific, to put it mildly.

I'm sure Ryan will be fine, he's a tough kid. These things do have a way of hanging around the subconscious, though.

Giving Thanks
I'm no Washington, but I do know a thing or two about giving thanks.

Yesterday at four in the afternoon I decided to go food shopping for the last-minute things necessary for a successful feast. I needed cranberry sauce, whole and jellied, turnips (I'm the only one who eats the stuff at my house), some gravy, milk, and some cream cheese. I never thought twice about the chances of all these things being available at my fingertips hours before a major holiday.

The shelves were stocked with food, fruit, fresh vegetables, thousands of cheeses, aisle after aisle of things, perishable and not.

I walked past the meat counter as the meat guy wheeled out a pallet full of turkeys. Fresh ones, frozen ones, big ones, little ones, they even had a duck and some geese.

If you took a person from the not so distant past and put him in my place yesterday, he might have thought he was in heaven. I thought of that after complaining to the grocery manager because there were no whole cranberries.

Thank you everybody who participates in our democracy, past, present, and future. It truly is amazing how we make this society work. It's nearly miraculous when you stop and think about it.

General Thanksgiving

By the PRESIDENT of the United States Of America

A PROCLAMATION

WHEREAS *it is the duty of all nations to acknowledge the providence of Almighty God, to obey His will, to be grateful for His benefits, and humbly to implore His protection and favour; and Whereas both Houses of Congress have, by their joint committee, requested me "to recommend to the people of the United States a DAY OF PUBLICK THANSGIVING and PRAYER, to be observed by acknowledging with grateful hearts the many and signal favors of Almighty God, especially by affording them an opportunity peaceably to establish a form of government for their safety and happiness:"*

NOW THEREFORE, *I do recommend and assign THURSDAY, the TWENTY-SIXTH DAY of NOVEMBER next, to be devoted by the people of these States to the service of that great and glorious Being who is the beneficent author of all the good that was, that is, or that will be; that we may then all unite in rendering unto Him our sincere and humble thanks for His kind care and protection of the people of this country previous to their becoming a nation; for the signal and manifold mercies and the favorable interpositions of His providence in the course and conclusion of the late war; for the great degree of tranquility, union, and plenty which we have since enjoyed;– for the peaceable and rational manner in which we have been enable to establish Constitutions of government for our safety and happiness, and particularly the national one now lately instituted;– for the civil and religious liberty with which we are blessed, and the means we have of acquiring and dissusing useful knowledge;– and, in general, for all the great and various favours which He has been pleased to confer upon us.*

And also, that we may then unite in most humbly offering our prayers and supplications to the great Lord and Ruler of Nations and beseech Him to pardon our national and other transgressions;– to enable us all, whether in publick or private stations, to perform our several and relative duties properly and punctually; to render our National Government a blessing to all the people by constantly being a Government of wife, just, and constitutional laws, discreetly and faithfully executed and obeyed; to protect and guide all sovereigns and nations (especially such as have shewn kindness unto us); and to bless them with good governments, peace, and concord; to promote the knowledge and practice of true religion and virtue, and the increase of science among them and us; and, generally to grant unto all mankind such a degree of temporal prosperity as he alone knows to be best.

GIVEN under my hand, at the city of New-York, the third day of October, in the year of our Lord, one thousand seven hundred and eighty-nine.

(signed) G. Washington

Black Friday

What exactly is Black Friday? You just know we're being taken advantage of when corporate America jumps on the urban myth bandwagon and starts to market a social phenomenon like Black Friday. I liked it better when we all knew that the day after Thanksgiving was shoppers' hell, no big ad campaign had to tell us but bargains were to be found if you looked. I actually passed a home improvement place today that was advertising "Black Friday Window Sale."

Sometimes I think we're on this planet to serve as revenue producers for other people. Then I remember yesterday, when things were quiet and I sat in my backyard smoking a cigar with my daughter's boyfriend and his dad talking about whatever came to mind. The girls were inside drinking wine and talking about whatever it is they talk about when they are left without their other halves. Simple, unplanned things like that make it all worthwhile. Nobody told us it was "Smoking Thanksgiving Eve" or anything, just three guys enjoying each other's company after a long, enjoyable holiday spent with our families.

I had a great day yesterday, and Black Friday is just another day, as far as I'm concerned.

Giddy-up

Patient: "I've waited weeks to see you; I'm hoping you can fix my back."

Doctor (surgeon actually): "Let's look at the films."

The doctor takes the MRI films from the manila envelope and places them onto the white viewing board. He doesn't miss a beat.

Doctor: "This is your spine. These are your vertebrae. This is your spinal fluid. These white areas are healthy discs.

These black areas are unhealthy discs. You have zero healthy discs in your entire lumbar spine."

Patient: "That can't be good."

Doctor: "It's not the end of the world. Pain management, core strengthening, and therapy you'll be all right."

Patient: "Will it return to normal?"

Doctor: "Normal for an eighty-year-old."

Patient: "What do you suggest?"

Doctor: "You're not a candidate for surgical repair, too much damage; I can't repair the entire lumbar spine. Live your life, live with the pain, and get on with things."

Patient: "Great."

There you have it. Three more weeks of "core strengthening" and back on the old horse. Not the answers I had hoped for.

Soon

Ryan stopped by yesterday, filled me in on some of what I've been missing (not) during my convalescence. I've got a couple of weeks of peace and quiet left before getting back into the thick of things. While my back has been healing, a lot of healing has happened in the old noggin as well. It is impossible to respond to call after call without some mental damage.

Teresa from Rescue 5 called last week. Among other things she mentioned a woman who jumped to her death at the major shopping mall. Another went the day after she called and a third two days ago. Seems the mall is as good a place as any to end it. Three suicides, one mall. The bodies splattered all over the parking garage.

Serenity now, for me anyway. Stay safe, and sane everybody.

There
Although I'm not always physically there, I never truly leave
Providence. My family began there, generations ago. I see
the skyline when I walk the shore near my home. I get my
pizza (Pizza Pier) on Wickenden Street and enjoy breakfast
there (Brickway) as well. I've stood for hours in front of
Picasso's masterpieces at the Rhode Island School of Design
Art Museum, and walked the same streets as Edgar Allen Poe
while contemplating my place on this earth. H. P. Lovecraft's
ghost joined me on some of these walks down Benefit Street,
I swear.

Roger Williams founded this place hundreds of years ago,
searching for a place free of religious persecution. I've spent
time relaxing in the park that bears his name. Last night I
attended *A Christmas Carol* at Trinity. Twelve of us enjoyed
the show, friends and family taking two rows of the theater,
strangers filling the rest. The ambiance and the humanity
one experiences when in the company of other, like-minded
people is contagious, and Peace on Earth seemed a possibility,
for a short time, anyway. Strangers and family came together,
captivated by the performers, filling the building with hope
and good cheer.

Outside, the Providence that has become waited.

Yesterday, three cops were shot and wounded during
a drug bust, shot by a reputed drug dealer in the West
End with a 9mm. Today, a sixteen-year-old succumbed to
gunshot wounds he got at a birthday party Sunday night.
Yesterday another sixteen-year-old from the South Side
was riddled with bullets. A few drive-bys, stabbings, and
beatings never made the headlines, but that doesn't mean
they didn't happen; there just wasn't room for the stories, or,
more likely, nobody cares.

Between the murders, MVAs, suicides, and accidents, the
body count since I injured my back is in the double digits. I

know it's my job, and I'm truly grateful to have it, but it's nice to spend time on the other side for a while. I stay in contact with a few people from the job. I'm sure they are not aware of it, just like I wasn't a few months ago, but the tension in their voices, and cynicism in their words, is disheartening.

Sorry for sounding like a broken record, but I'm shocked at the difference I feel from then to now. What worries me is now is about to happen, and I'm not sure if I'm ready, or more accurately, willing.

The Gift
Some, not all, have been given a gift worth much more than anything that comes from a store. I am one of those fortunates. Without asking, wishing for, or even realizing I had it until well into my adulthood, the ability to work as a firefighter/ EMT was bestowed upon me. This was the first gift; the next came with a little work. I had to put those gifts into action, first by learning, then by finding a place to put this gift to use. Fortunately for me, that place is the Providence Fire Department.

Through all the contractual squabbles, petty rivalries between firefighters and rescue people, and relentless calls, I can't think of anything I would rather have. Friendships with hundreds of people have been made possible because of this gift, doctors, nurses, patients, security, cops, teachers . . . the list is long. A whole world is open to me because of what I do. Who I am opens that world even further, and who I am is a direct result of the gift that was given to me.

People I don't know call 911 and wait, their anxiety high, fear, uncertainty, and despair wait for me to show up. That I can respond, and alleviate some of that, is truly a miracle, one I don't take lightly. It is something worth remembering during the toughest shifts. However bad we have it, the people on the other end of the phone usually have it worse. And I help them. For that opportunity I am thankful.

This is the season for giving. For all the giving I do, I honestly believe I have received far more.

The Core

Six weeks of core strengthening, dieting, glucosamine, and endurance training have led me to this:

"You're all done."

"Done, you say? Never!"

Two doctors, my primary physician and the orthopedic specialist, have essentially ended my career as a rescue lieutenant. But, I ask, "Have you seen these abs?"

I'll be back on the truck, I swear.

Light duty starts Monday, 0700 hrs. I can hardly wait.

One Step at a Time

> *This Winter harsh and cruel will not change much for us*
> *it is a time to be together, a time for closeness and of warmth,*
> *a time to renew strength to start with vigour our battle.*
>
> *Susie Hemingway*

Battles are fought every day, courageous, relentless, and deadly. Inside the homes we pass, the minds of the people we greet and in the hospitals and nursing homes where people spend their last days, struggles larger than many of us can imagine take place. Suffering is handled with dignity and grace. Despair hidden behind brave faces whose true pain is kept hidden, except for those closest, and sometimes, even from them.

There is a true hero who walks alongside of me, battling multiple sclerosis, helped by a cane, stumbling, frustrated, and in pain. Our battle marches on, relentless.

I'll heal. I'll walk, maybe swagger. I'll lift and carry, perhaps without the gusto I once had, but I'll pull my weight. My bones will creak and muscles will ache, but I'll go on. So will Cheryl. One step at a time.

Another battle begins. I'll be Lieutenant Morse again. But I'll always be Mrs. Morse's husband.

AFTERWORD

I returned to full duty and managed to get through nearly four more years, one run at a time. Without help from the people I work with I never would have made it. Seldom did I carry a patient during that time; firefighters would push me out of the way and do the heavy lifting. I wish I could have gone on doing what I love forever. My mind was able, my body had other plans.

So now I write about the things I did. Sometimes I miss being able to do it. Most of the time I am content knowing that during the time I spent responding to other people's emergencies, I did my damndest.

Thanks for reading.